STUDENT WORKBOOK
to accompany

Mosby's Guide to
PHYSICAL
EXAMINATION

THIRD EDITION

SEIDEL • BALL • DAINS • BENEDICT

MINDI MILLER, R.N., Ph. D.

Faculty
Department of
Human Performance and Health Sciences
Rice University
Houston, Texas

Nursing Diagnosis and Considerations content
contributed by

NANCY WATSON, R.N., M.S.N.

Deaconess Medical Center
St. Louis, Missouri

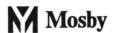 Mosby

St. Louis Baltimore Boston Carlsbad Chicago Naples New York Philadelphia Portland
London Madrid Mexico City Singapore Sydney Tokyo Toronto Wiesbaden

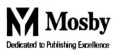
Mosby
Dedicated to Publishing Excellence

A Times Mirror Company

Publisher: Nancy L. Coon
Editor: Sally Schrefer
Developmental Editors: Penny Rudolph and Gail Brower
Project Manager: Patricia Tannian
Senior Production Editor: Ann E. Rogers
Senior Book Designer: Gail Morey Hudson
Cover Designer: Teresa Breckwoldt
Manufacturing Supervisor: Kathy Grone

THIRD EDITION

Printed in the United States of America

Printing/binding by Plus Communications

Mosby–Year Book, Inc.
11830 Westline Industrial Drive
St. Louis, Missouri 63146

International Standard Book Number ISBN 0-8151-6210-3

94 95 96 97 98 / 9 8 7 6 5 4 3 2 1

Contributors

MONA RAE MERRYMAN, R.N., B.S.N., B.A., C.C.R.N.

Critical Care Clinician
Long Beach, California
Adjunct Faculty
Mt. San Antonio College
Walnut, California

CAROL A. NORMAN, R.N., M. Ed., M.S.N.

Nursing Faculty
North Harris College
Houston, Texas

HELEN M. STARKWEATHER, R.N., M.S.N.

Nursing Instructor
North Harris College
Houston, Texas

Reviewers

JANE W. BALL, R.N., C.P.N.P., Dr. PH.

Manager, Pediatric Emergency Education and Research Center
Children's National Medical Center
Washington, D. C.

DIANNE G. COPENHAVER, B.S.N., M.S., Ph. D.

Associate Professor of Nursing
Coppin State College
Baltimore, Maryland

JOYCE E. DAINS, R.N., Dr. P.H., J.D.

Former Associate Professor, School of Nursing
The University of Texas–Houston Health Science Center
Houston, Texas

Preface

This workbook is divided into three sections. Part I presents questions and learning exercises for each chapter of *Mosby's Guide to Physical Examination*. The workbook chapters give learning objectives, a learning focus, and activities that assess and facilitate student comprehension. At the end of each workbook chapter are questions concerning nursing considerations. Section II must be studied in order to complete these questions.

Part II addresses nursing considerations. This content centers on the nursing process. Nursing diagnoses derived from physical examination findings are discussed. Each chapter of Section II includes data on the health history, physical assessment, and diagnostic procedures. The definition for each nursing diagnosis, as well as the related factors and defining characteristics, including subjective and objective data, are delineated. Frequent case studies are presented in this section.

Part III includes helpful information related to examination findings. The first tool is an outline of expected adult findings. The second reference is documentation of findings from a history and physical examination for "M.L.," a fictional person. Because this hypothetical examination is a general check-up, a chief complaint is not stated. A general appraisal is followed by a description of findings from each system.

Mindi Miller

Contents

How to Use This Workbook

LEARNING OBJECTIVES

This workbook follows a clear, simple format. Chapter learning objectives are stated at the beginning of each chapter. These objectives are placed under headings that reflect their focus. Chapter objectives are cognitive objectives that relate to didactic content.

DIRECTIONS FOR LEARNING ACTIVITIES

Pay particular attention to the directions below, since directions are *not* included within the workbook. Five standard question formats are used, and instructions for completing these recurrent question types are as follows.

Multiple Choice

Each multiple choice question has only *one* best answer. The answer choices are usually given in alphabetic or chronologic order. Select one answer per question.

SAMPLE:

Which one of the following history sections briefly states the reason why the patient seeks health care?

A. Chief complaint
B. Family history
C. Past medical history
D. Systems review

(*Answer:* A, Chief complaint)

Matching

Pair the items on the right with those on the left. Only *one* answer is used in each blank. *All* answers should be used.

SAMPLE:

Definition
_____ 1. Aunt T. has migraines.
_____ 2. "I have head pain."
_____ 3. Works in factory.

History Structure
A. Chief complaint
B. Family history
C. Personal history

(*Answers:* 1. B, Family history; 2. A, Chief complaint; 3. C, Personal history)

Modified Matching

Match the terms in the right hand column with those on the left. Some terms will be used more than once. If an abbreviation for the term is given, write that in the blank to save time.

SAMPLE:

Body Organs and Systems

_____ 1. Circulatory
_____ 2. Thymus
_____ 3. Respiratory
_____ 4. Brain

Specialized Tissues

G = General
L = Lymphoid
N = Neural

(*Answers:* 1. G, 2. L, 3. G, 4. N, 5. N, 6. G)

TRUE or Corrected Statement

If the statement is true, write "TRUE" in the space provided. If the statement is false, change the underlined words to make it true. You do *not* need to write the word "false." Write as many words as needed to make the statement true, but replace only the underlined words. The number of false words and your corrected statement do not have to match word for word.

SAMPLES:

_____ 1. Mobility is greatest at level L1-5.
_____ 2. Culture is a shared set of values.
_____ 3. Feinstein calls "pain" the iatrophic stimulus that causes patients to seek health care.

(*Answers:* 1. C5-7; 2. TRUE; 3. TRUE.)

Completion

Completion exercises involve short answers to questions. Lined spaces are allocated for your answers.

SAMPLE:

What is meant by "beneficence"?

_____

_____

(*Answer:* The care provider's need to do good for the patient.)

GUIDELINES

Self-assessment will be more accurate and learning will be better facilitated if you follow the seven steps below.

1. Read a chapter from the textbook (*Mosby's Guide to Physical Examination*) and make notes on the content.
2. Read the corresponding chapter on nursing considerations and nursing diagnoses in Part II of this workbook.
3. Review available videotapes and interactive videodiscs.
4. Then, relying only on memory, complete as many of the learning activities in the workbook chapter as possible.
5. Re-read pages from the textbook or Part II of this workbook that are associated with any learning activity you left undone.
6. Complete the workbook chapter.
7. Check your answers with your instructor.

The workbook exercises have been developed to correspond with the chapter learning objectives. Headings within the objectives, such as "Anatomy and Physioloy," are repeated in the learning activities sections. If you successfully complete a section but still have additional questions, review the textbook pages or other learning resources, such as available videotapes, once again.

NOTE: Textbook page numbers that correspond to most of the workbook questions are listed at the back of this workbook. Page numbers for Nursing Considerations questions are omitted, since content relating to these questions is not found in the textbook. See Part II of this workbook to research answers for nursing considerations questions.

Part I
STUDENT WORKBOOK EXERCISES

STUDENT WORKBOOK EXERCISE

<table>
<tr><td>

Chapter 1
</td><td>

The History and Interviewing Process
</td></tr>
</table>

LEARNING OBJECTIVES

After (1) reading the textbook chapter, pages 1–33, (2) studying the introduction and overview of the nursing process in Part II of this workbook, and (3) completing the following questions, students should be able to:

COMMUNICATION WITH PATIENTS

1. Recognize ethical considerations in patient–examiner relationships.
2. Describe factors that enhance communication.
3. Identify situations that precipitate feelings of tension between interviewers and patients.
4. Delineate feelings and behaviors that facilitate or impede the interviewing process.
5. Recognize environments that facilitate or impede information gathering.
6. Compare age and condition variations in communication relevant to the interviewing process.

HISTORY

7. Identify the appropriate structure of the history.
8. Select relevant questions for history taking.
9. Apply general guidelines and assessment techniques for conducting a history.
10. Organize data according to a clinical history outline.
11. Revise history taking to acommodate age and condition variations.

NURSING CONSIDERATIONS

12. Explain the nursing process.
13. Delineate the five steps of the nursing process.
14. Describe the three components of a comprehensive database.

Explain the following terms:

15. Defining characteristics
16. Health assessments
17. Nursing diagnosis
18. Objective data/findings
19. Patient database
20. Physical assessment
21. Physical examination
22. Related factors
23. Sign
24. Subjective data/findings
25. Symptom

STUDY FOCUS

Interviewing skills must be developed so that health care providers will interpret rather than misinterpret information about a patient's health status. Obtaining a history involves the collection of data relevant to a patient's past, present, and potential health problems. By completing the following exercises, you will review factors that facilitate communication, enhance your interviewing skills, and optimize your history–taking abilities.

LEARNING ACTIVITIES

COMMUNICATION WITH PATIENTS

Matching

Definition	Term
_____ 1. Care giver's desire to not harm the patient	A. Autonomy
_____ 2. Care giver's need to help the patient	B. Beneficence
_____ 3. General need to use resources for community well–being	C. Nonmaleficence
_____ 4. Patient's need for self determination	D. Utilitarianism

Completion

5. List at least four factors that enhance your skills as a communicator.
   A. _____
   B. _____
   C. _____
   D. _____

6. Describe in the space provided at least one situation in which you were interviewed by a health care giver and found yourself feeling tense.

   _____
   _____
   _____

Patient Behavior	Examiner Behavior That May Decrease Tension
7. Silence	7.A. _____
	B. _____
8. Crying	8.A. _____
	B. _____
9. Seduction	9.A. _____
	B. _____
10. Anger	10.A _____
	B. _____
11. Dissemblance	11.A. _____
	B. _____

Age or Condition	Techniques That May Enhance Communication
12. Children	12.A. _____
	B. _____
13. Older adults	13.A. _____
	B. _____
14. Handicapped persons	14.A. _____
	B. _____

Multiple Choice

15. Which person would be more likely to promote accurate and confidential interpretations for a non–English speaking patient?
    A. Clergy
    B. Family member
    C. Housekeeper
    D. Medical personnel

16. The assessment of all verbal and nonverbal communication is best described as:
    A. cognitive examination.
    B. intelligent repose.
    C. open–ended assessment.
    D. reflective thinking.

17. Interviewers should identify and assess their own feelings, such as hostility and prejudice, in order to:
    A. avoid inappropriate behavior.
    B. explain their biases to patients.
    C. express their idiosyncracies.
    D. promote self awareness.

Situation: You are interviewing Ms. N. who appears distressed. She states that she is very upset about the reoccurrence of her skin rash. Ms. N. verbalizes compliance with her previous skin treatment plan.

18. Your most appropriate response would be to:
    A. acknowledge her feelings and proceed with her history.
    B. ask "yes" and "no" questions about her skin condition.
    C. ignore her inappropriate expressions of anger.
    D. tell her that she is getting upset over nothing.

Situation: During an interview with a client, he describes abdominal pain that often awakens him at night.

19. Which of the following responses facilitates the interviewing process?
    A. Constipation can cause abdominal pain.
    B. Do you need a sleeping medication?
    C. Pain is always worse at night.
    D. Tell me what you mean by "often."

20. You should take time to ask patients about their lifestyle and values in order to:
    A. assess their economic status and ability to pay.
    B. document their sexuality and any deviations from normal.
    C. identify cultural factors pertinent to their health care.
    D. make small talk until the patient feels comfortable.

Situation: When taking a client's history, you are asked questions about your personal life.

21. What is the best response to facilitate the interviewing process?
    A. Answer briefly and then refocus to the patient's history.
    B. Give as much detail as possible about the asked information.
    C. Ignore the question and continue with the patient's history.
    D. Tell the patient that you cannot answer personal questions.

22. When you repeat a patient's answer, you are trying to:
    A. confirm an accurate understanding.
    B. discourage patient anger or hostility.
    C. teach the patient new medical terms.
    D. test the patient's knowledge.

HISTORY

Matching

	Description	*Term*
_____	23. Brief description of perceived problem	A. Chief complaint
_____	24. Chronological course of events	B. Family history
_____	25. Organized physiologic data	C. Medical history
_____	26. Pedigree diagram	D. Present problem
_____	27. Previous childhood and adult illnesses	E. Systems review

Completion

28. Describe five types of questions that should be asked about the patient's present illness.

    A. _____

    B. _____

    C. _____

    D. _____

    E. _____

29. List at least six developmental milestones that are part of a preschool child's history.
    Age when child was able to:

    A. _____

    B. _____

    C. _____

    D. _____

    E. _____

    F. _____

30. Explain why health care providers should avoid using jargon, arcane, and pejorative words.

    _____

    _____

    _____

TRUE or Corrected Statement

_____ 31. The <u>iatrotropic stimulus</u> refers to the reason why a patient seeks health care.

_____ 32. Before concluding an interview, the examiner should <u>encourage patient questions</u>.

_____ 33. A <u>PACE Assessment</u> is used to evaluate a patient's alcohol consumption.

_____ 34. About <u>two percent</u> of patients will have homosexual or bisexual preferences.

_____ 35. The events and symptoms described by the patient should be placed in the record <u>in any sequence</u> within the present problem section.

_____ 36. Childhood and major adult illnesses should be recorded in the <u>family history section</u>.

_____ 37. The <u>review of systems</u> section for women should include data on menses, pregnancies, and breast health.

_____ 38. For pregnant women, data about their LMP, PNMP, and EDC belong in the <u>past medical history</u> section.

_____ 39. A survey of mobility and activities of daily living is part of a <u>social history</u>.

_____ 40. Catastrophic illness is more apt to be a problem among <u>the elderly</u> than among other ages.

NURSING CONSIDERATIONS

Matching

Techniques

_____ 41. Evaluation of body and functional abilities

_____ 42. History, examination and diagnostic data

_____ 43. Holistic approach assessing mind, body and spirit

_____ 44. Logical, five step problem solving tool

_____ 45. Methods used to collect only objective data

Terms

A. Health Assessment

B. Nursing Process

C. Patient Data Base

D. Physical Assessment

E. Physical Examination

Nursing Process

_____ 46. Analysis of data to identify patient problems and needs

_____ 47. Assessment of intervention effectiveness

_____ 48. Care given and interventions done

_____ 49. Goal setting and anticipated interventions

_____ 50. Systematic, comprehensive data collection

Terms

A. Assessment

B. Evaluation

C. Implementation

D. Nursing Diagnosis

E. Plan

Findings

_____ 51. Abnormal finding

_____ 52. Measurable finding

_____ 53. Patient's statements

_____ 54. Risks and etiologies

_____ 55. Signs

_____ 56. Symptoms

Definitions

A. Defining characteristics

B. Manifestation of problem

C. Objective information

D. Patient's feelings

E. Related factors

F. Subjective information

Multiple Choice

57. The nursing process combines all the skills of:
    A. abstract reasoning.
    B. critical thinking.
    C. diagnostic evaluation.
    D. Freudian analysis.

58. The technique used for problem solving and assisting the nurse with clinical decision making is the:
    A. concrete thinking method.
    B. cultural sensitivity scale.
    C. nursing process.
    D. patient database.

59. Health history information, examination findings, and diagnostic studies are data belonging in the patient's:
    A. data base.
    B. holistic plan.
    C. status report.
    D. temporary file.

60. The primary source of data that is often the best source of information comes from:
    A. diagnostic studies.
    B. family members.
    C. medical records.
    D. patients themselves.

Chapter 2

Cultural Awareness

STUDY FOCUS

Culturally related terms are complex by definition and often interrelated. For practical purposes, culture is described in very general ways for the purpose of implying group characteristics. When studying this chapter, review the basic beliefs, behaviors, and health practices of individuals who share environments and values.

LEARNING ACTIVITIES

GENERAL CULTURAL CONCEPTS

Multiple Choice

1. An integral part of the overall effort to respond well to a person in need is:
   A. cultural awareness.
   B. ethnocentric bias.
   C. political correctness.
   D. racial alertness.

2. An example of a cultural characteristic is:
   A. gender type.
   B. habitual drinking.
   C. nose size.
   D. shared belief.

3. A stereotypic behavior that regulates situational actions is a/an:
   A. ethnos.
   B. rite.
   C. ritual.
   D. value.

4. In the United States, morbidity and mortality rates are highest among:
   A. low economic groups.
   B. middle class women.
   C. Roman catholic priests.
   D. white collar professionals.

5. Which one of the following is a correct statement that shows an interrelationship between culture and societal conditions?
   A. College graduates tend to live longer than high school dropouts.
   B. Individuals with the same skin color have similar mortality rates.
   C. Invasive cardiac procedures are performed more often on blacks than on whites.
   D. Morbidity rates are greater among individuals with high incomes.

Matching

	Definition	*Term*
_____	6. Formal, religious, or other ceremonial acts	A. Culture
		B. Custom
_____	7. Habitual activity passed along by family members	C. Rite
		D. Ritual
_____	8. Reflects the whole of human behavior	
_____	9. Regulating behavior used in different situations	

	Definition	*Term*
_____	10. Accepts a particular cultural identity	A. Acculturation
_____	11. Believes own culture is superior	B. Enculturation
_____	12. Inflexible generalization about a group	C. Ethnocentric
_____	13. Sheds one culture and assumes another culture	D. Stereotype

	Definition	*Term*
_____	14. Behavior approved by group standards	A. Ethnos
_____	15. Desirable or undesirable group ideals and behavior	B. Minority
		C. Norm
_____	16. Group with same origin and culture	D. Race
_____	17. Physical characteristic not based on culture	E. Value
_____	18. Population different than this group	

TRUE or Corrected Statement

_____ 19. The root of social, political, and economic tragedy often stems from <u>cultural blurring</u>.

_____ 20. Whenever practical, a patient's health perceptions should be <u>changed</u>.

_____ 21. "How bad is your sickness?" is a question aimed at discovering the patient's <u>culture</u>.

Matching

Time Orientation	*Cultural Group*
_____ 22. Accepts each day as it comes	A. Dominant American
_____ 23. Continues meaningful past traditions	B. Eastern Asian
_____ 24. Places high value on change	C. Hispanic, Black, Native American

Activity Orientation	*Cultural Group*
_____ 25. Accomplishments measured by external standards	A. Dominant American
_____ 26. Emphasizes holistic self development	B. Eastern Asian
_____ 27. Spontaneous self expression	C. Hispanic, Black, Native American

Human-Nature Orientation	*Cultural Group*
_____ 28. Humans are neither good nor evil	A. Dominant American
_____ 29. Humans are masters over nature	B. Eastern Asian, Native American
_____ 30. Humans have little control over destiny	C. Hispanic, Black

Relational Orientation	*Cultural Group*
_____ 31. Collateral relationships	A. Dominant American
_____ 32. Individualistic and impersonal relationships	B. Eastern Asian
_____ 33. Lineal relationships	C. Hispanic, Black, North American

CULTURE AND HEALTH CARE

Matching

Infant Baptism Practices	*Religion*
_____ 34. Done 8-40 days after birth	A. Anglican-Episcopal
_____ 35. Mandatory for all infants	B. Eastern Orthodox
_____ 36. Not really necessary	C. Hindu
_____ 37. Only living children baptized soon after birth	D. Lutheran
_____ 38. Priest baptism only	E. Orthodox Presbyterian
_____ 39. Sprinkling done	F. Russian Orthodox
_____ 40. Water placed into deceased child's mouth	G. Unitarian Universalist

Multiple Choice

41. Which cultural group believes that evil is removed by purification?
    A. Filipino
    B. Haitian
    C. Japanese
    D. Vietnamese

42. Which cultural group uses outside agencies and fortune tellers to treat the ill?
    A. Filipino
    B. Haitian
    C. Japanese
    D. Vietnamese

43. The use of condiments, such as monosodium glutamate to promote health, is predominately practiced by:
    A. Asian American Chinese
    B. Cuban Americans
    C. Hispanic and Mexican Americans
    D. Native Americans

44. A variety of treatment options, such as traditional medicine, santeros, and public health services are used by:
    A. Asian American Chinese
    B. Cuban Americans
    C. Hispanic and Mexican Americans
    D. Native Americans

45. The use of prayer, self-care, voodoo and folk medicine is most prevalent in:
    A. African Americans
    B. Haitians
    C. Puerto Ricans
    D. Native Americans

46. Singers that cure by the power of their songs are often used by:
    A. African Americans
    B. Haitians
    C. Puerto Ricans
    D. Native Americans

Completion

47. Describe at least two different forms of communication that are culturally determined.

    A. _____

    B. _____

48. Compose at least one question that you could ask patients concerning each of the following cultural assessment categories.

    A. HEALTH BELIEFS AND PRACTICES:_____

    _____

    B. RELIGIOUS AND RITUAL INFLUENCES: _____

    _____

    C. LANGUAGE AND COMMUNICATION:_____

    _____

    D. PARENTING AND FAMILY ASPECTS: _____

    _____

    E. DIETARY PRACTICES: _____

    _____

TRUE or Corrected Statement

_____ 49. A food that may be considered "hot" is <u>chocolate</u>.

_____ 50. Milk of magnesia is considered to be a <u>lukewarm herb</u>.

_____ 51. An <u>earache</u> is an example of a "hot" symptom or condition.

_____ 52. <u>Cancer</u> is an example of a "cold" condition.

_____ 53. <u>Penicillin</u> is considered to be a "hot" medicine.

_____ 54. <u>Honey</u> is an example of a "cold" food.

_____ 55. <u>Garlic</u> is considered a "cold" herb.

_____ 56. There tends to be a correlation between receiving <u>prenatal care</u> and seeking infant inoculations.

_____ 57. Western medicine is replete with <u>plants and herbs</u>.

_____ 58. Fathers becoming involved with child care is an example of an <u>ethnic stability</u>.

Multiple Choice

Situation: *You are taking care of an elderly gentleman from Fiji. After reading about Fiji, you learn that raising your arms while talking may be perceived as impolite. You also learn that talking with your arms folded in front of you may be considered respectful.*

59. While talking with your patient, you would:
    A. cross your arms over your chest.
    B. don't move at all when speaking.
    C. hold your hands behind your back.
    D. raise only one hand when speaking.

Situation: *You are conducting a routine examination on a young, obese woman raised in Panama. She has been trying to conceive for a few months. You know that individuals from Panama may view body fat as a sign of good health and fertility.*

60. Your best initial response would be to say:
    A. "I think you should change your diet and lose weight."
    B. "What kind of things do you usually eat and drink?"
    C. "What do you think would help you achieve pregnancy?"
    D. "You may need to undergo extensive fertility tests."

Chapter 3

Examination Techniques and Equipment

STUDY FOCUS

All examination techniques must be performed accurately and safely. The following questions relate to universal precautions and standard examination techniques. The proper use of instrumentation to achieve accurate findings is reviewed.

16

LEARNING ACTIVITIES

EXAMINATION TECHNIQUES

TRUE or Corrected Statement

_____ 1. <u>Sterilization</u> is the most essential method for preventing the spread of infection.

_____ 2. Masks, eyewear, or face shields should be worn during <u>venous punctures</u>.

_____ 3. Some individuals perceive <u>direct touch</u> as an invasion of privacy.

_____ 4. North American middle class groups generally perceive <u>eye contact</u> as an important aspect of communication.

_____ 5. Tangential lighting enhances observation of <u>texture</u>.

_____ 6. Finger pressure is about <u>1cm</u> during deep palpation.

_____ 7. The <u>dorsal</u> surface of the examiner's hand is best for palpating vibration.

_____ 8. The more dense the medium, the <u>quieter</u> the percussion tone.

_____ 9. <u>Tympany</u> is the loudest percussion sound.

_____ 10. <u>Dullness</u> is the quietest percussion sound.

Modified Matching

Palpation Finding

_____ 11. Position
_____ 12. Vibration
_____ 13. Texture
_____ 14. Size
_____ 15. Temperature
_____ 16. Masses
_____ 17. Fluid
_____ 18. Crepitus

Anatomy

D = Dorsal surface of hands
P = Palmar surface of fingers
U = Ulnar surface of hands

Matching

Media

_____ 19. Emphysematous lungs
_____ 20. Gastric bubble
_____ 21. Healthy lung
_____ 22. Liver or spleen
_____ 23. Muscle

Percussion Tone

D = Dullness
F = Flatness
H = Hyperresonance
R = Resonance
T = Tympany

Completion

24. List at least four guidelines for inspecting the body.

    A. _____

    B. _____

    C. _____

    D. _____

25. Describe in the space provided the techniques of direct and indirect percussion.

    _____

    _____

    _____

    _____

    _____

Multiple Choice

26. What is the usual sequence of examination procedures?
    A. Auscultation, inspection, palpation, percussion
    B. Inspection, palpation, percussion, auscultation
    C. Inspection, percussion, auscultation, palpation
    D. Palpation, percussion, auscultation, inspection

    Situation: Ms. J. is admitted with draining abdominal fistulas. She is also incontinent. Ms. J. is very thin. She appears oriented and states that she is very modest.

27. Which one of the following is the most important initial procedure?
    A. Describe how you will maintain privacy
    B. Establish universal precautions
    C. Orient the patient to the room
    D. Remove and change her diapers

28. What part of the examiner's hand should be used for detecting tenderness of the liver, gallbladder, or kidneys?
    A. Closed fist
    B. Finger tips
    C. Palmar surface
    D. Ulnar aspect

29. Information from resonance sounds heard without the aid of a stethoscope is obtained by performing:
    A. auscultation.
    B. inspection.
    C. palpation.
    D. percussion.

30. Focused visual attention obtains data from:
    A. auscultation.
    B. inspection.
    C. palpation.
    D. percussion.

INSTRUMENTATION

Completion

31. Delineate at least four steps that you would take to promote an accurate blood pressure reading.
    A. _____
    _____
    B. _____
    _____
    C. _____
    _____
    D. _____
    _____

32. State at least one advantage and one disadvantage that may be associated with the use of a tympanic membrane thermometer.
    A. ADVANTAGE: _____
    _____
    B. DISADVANTAGE: _____
    _____

33. Describe at least four stethoscope characteristics that promote accurate acoustic results.
    A. _____
    _____
    B. _____
    _____
    C. _____
    _____
    D. _____
    _____

Multiple Choice

34. For children, a blood pressure cuff should be:
    A. double the child's neck size.
    B. equal to the limb length.
    C. the same width as the limb circumference.
    D. two thirds of the upper arm or thigh.

35. Slow inflation of the blood pressure cuff will promote:
    A. accurate readings.
    B. arterial leaps.
    C. capillary refill.
    D. venous congestion.

36. An instrument used to detect fetal heart tones and blood pressure sounds in obese persons and patients in shock is the:
    A. doppler.
    B. episcope.
    C. goniometer.
    D. sphygmomanometer.

37. Rotating the ophthalmoscope lens clockwise and counterclockwise can compensate for which condition in either the examiner or the patient?
    A. Amblyopia
    B. Astigmatism
    C. Hyperopia
    D. Strabismus

38. Which instrument uses a one-way mirror to help detect a patient's subtle eye movements?
    A. Episcope
    B. Ophthalmoscope
    C. Otoscope
    D. Strabismoscope

39. What instrument may be used if a nasal speculum is not available?
    A. Goniometer
    B. Hemostat
    C. Neurologic brush
    D. Otoscope

40. Which one of the following is a graphic representation of the change in compliance of the middle ear system as air pressure is varied?
    A. Electrogram
    B. Sphygmogram
    C. Thermogram
    D. Tympanogram

41. You may activate a tuning fork by tapping the prongs against your:
    A. chest.
    B. elbow.
    C. knuckles.
    D. wrist.

42. When examining children, what can you use as a reflex hammer?
    A. Cotton tip
    B. Examiner's finger
    C. Tongue blade
    D. Tuning fork

43. What are Graves and Pederson instruments that contain blades and thumbscrews?
    A. Lighting devices
    B. Joint goniometers
    C. Skinfold calipers
    D. Vaginal specula

44. What are Lange and Herpenden instruments?
    A. Lighting devices
    B. Joint goniometers
    C. Skinfold calipers
    D. Vaginal specula

Matching

	Examination Use	*Aperture*
_____	45. Estimating fundal lesion size	A. Grid
_____	46. Examining anterior eye	B. Red–free filter
_____	47. Viewing small pupils	C. Small aperture
_____	48. Viewing vessel changtes in disc	D. Slit

Statement

_____ 49. For auditory evaulation
_____ 50. Fork vibrates 512 cycles per second
_____ 51. Greatest sensitivity to vibration
_____ 52. Range of normal speech

Frequency

A. 100-400 Hz
B. 512 Hz
C. 500-1000 Hz
D. 300-3000 Hz

Statement

_____ 53. Epiluminescence microscopy
_____ 54. Shows presence of fungi
_____ 55. Strong light with narrow beam
_____ 56. Used with a penlight

Equipment

A. Episcope
B. Nasal speculum
C. Transilluminator
D. Wood's lamp

Completion

57. In the space provided, describe how you would test a patient's near vision if you didn't have a Rosenbaum or Jaeger chart.

_____

_____

_____

58. List three measurements taken with a tape measure.

A. _____

B. _____

C. _____

59. List three media that transmit light in a body cavity.

A. _____

B. _____

C. _____

60. In the space provided, describe differences in operation of plastic and metal vaginal specula.

_____

_____

_____

Chapter 4

Growth and Measurement

LEARNING OBJECTIVES

After (1) reading the textbook chapter, pages 84–130, (2) studying nursing considerations for Nutrition in Part II of this workbook, and (3) completing the following questions, students should be able to:

ANATOMY AND PHYSIOLOGY

1. Recognize anatomic and physiologic factors influencing growth.
2. Identify life phase variations in organ and tissue growth and developmental measurements.

HISTORY

3. Select patient information relevant to the present problem data of a growth and development history.
4. Gather personal and social history data pertinent to a patient's growth and development assessment.
5. Collect past medical and family data relevant to a growth and development history.

EXAMINATION AND FINDINGS

6. Indicate appropriate equipment and techniques for measuring growth and development.
7. Assess expected findings relevant to growth and development throughout the life cycle.
8. Appraise variations suggesting potential disorders and abnormalities of growth and development throughout the life cycle.

NURSING CONSIDERATIONS

9. Assess nutritional factors associated with growth and measurement.
10. Evaluate cultural factors pertinent to growth and measurement.
11. Apply critical thinking towards analyzing nursing considerations while measuring growth and development.
12. Formulate appropriate nursing diagnoses after completing a growth and development assessment.

STUDY FOCUS

There are many life cycle changes that occur in the anatomy and physiology of humans. These workbook questions focus on expected findings during the growth process, and data that will alert you to actual or potential health problems. Physical and physiologic measurements are crucial to the interpretation of growth and well being throughout the life cycle.

LEARNING ACTIVITIES

ANATOMY AND PHYSIOLOGY

Multiple Choice

1. What hormone stimulates DNA synthesis during adulthood?
   A. Androgen
   B. Growth hormone
   C. Sex hormone
   D. Thyroxin

2. Developmental changes seen during puberty are caused by the interaction of the gonads, the hypothalamus, and the:
   A. parathyroid gland.
   B. pituitary gland.
   C. thymus gland.
   D. thyroid gland.

3. Lymphatic tissues are at their peak around age:
   A. 6 months.
   B. 6 years.
   C. 12 years.
   D. 20 years.

4. Eighty percent of brain growth is completed by age:
   A. 1 year
   B. 2 years.
   C. 4 years.
   D. 7 years.

5. Skeletal growth is complete when the epiphyses of the long bones have:
   A. completely fused.
   B. disappeared.
   C. doubled in size.
   D. grown apart.

6. During gestational weeks 6 and 7, what embryonic structures are most sensitive to teratogens?
   A. Arms and legs
   B. Eyes and forehead
   C. Heart and nervous system
   D. Teeth and palate

7. Skeletal mass and organ systems double in size during:
   A. adolescence.
   B. infancy.
   C. menopause.
   D. pregnancy.

8. During pregnancy, what accounts for 5 to 10 pounds of the mother's total weight gain?
   A. Amniotic fluid
   B. Blood volume
   C. Fetus
   D. Placenta

9. Thinning of the intervertebral disks resulting in kyphosis is most likely to occur:
   A. after birth.
   B. at puberty.
   C. during pregnancy.
   D. with aging.

10. Between ages 30 and 80 years, muscle mass decreases about:
    A. 10% to 20%
    B. 21% to 29%
    C. 30% to 40%
    D. 41% to 50%

HISTORY

Matching

	Data Obtained from Patient	*Most Appropriate History Section*
_____	11. Gastric or renal illness	A. Family
_____	12. Recent change in body proportion	B. Past medical
_____	13. Statute or puberty disorder	C. Personal/social
_____	14. Usual nutritional habits	D. Present problem

	Data Obtained During History	*Most Pertinent Life Cycle*
_____	15. Achieving developmental milestones	A. Children and adolescents
_____	16. Activities of daily living	B. Infants and toddlers
_____	17. Age of menarche	C. Older adults
_____	18. Date of last menses	D. Pregnant women

Completion

19. Describe four pieces of information that may suggest body proportion or fat distribution changes. Explain the relevance of these findings.

A. _____

B. _____

C. _____

D. _____

Relevance: _____

_____

20. List at least two items that should be obtained as part of a patient's nutritional history.

A. _____

B. _____

21. State two anthropometric measurements that belong in a patient's history.

A. _____

B. _____

EXAMINATION AND FINDINGS

Completion

22. In the space provided, explain how you would determine the site of a triceps skinfold thickness measurement.

_____

_____

_____

_____

Situation: *Ms. L., age 45, has a height of 165 cm. She has an appropriate weight of 65 kg, and her triceps skinfold measurement is 20 mm.*

23. What do you know about her frame size and growth?

_____

_____

_____

_____

24. Describe in the space provided how you would determine height velocity in a child.

_____

_____

_____

_____

Situation: *Baby Mike is a 1–day–old neonate. You are performing a physical assessment and observe the following findings:*

   Measurements:
Birth weight 3250 gm; length 47.5 cm
Head circumference 33.0 cm
Chest circumference 32.0 cm
Neuromuscular maturity rating: Score of 16:
3 points for posture, arm recoil, scarf sign, and heel to ear
2 points for square window and popliteal angle
Appearance:
Half of his back devoid of lanugo; 3 to 4 mm areola diameter
Pale pink skin with a few visible blood vessels
Firm pinna with instant recoil
Plantar creases over entire heel
Testes descended with moderate rugae

25. Circle the boxes on the Newborn Maturity Rating and Classification form to indicate Mike's correct:
    A. neuromuscular maturity;
    B. physical maturity; and
    C. maturity score and gestational age.

26. Use circles to plot Mike's measurements on the graphs for:
    A. length;
    B. weight; and
    C. head circumference.

27. Mike's plotted percentile is around:

_____

28. How would you interpret the meaning of Mike's percentile and gestation?

_____

_____

_____

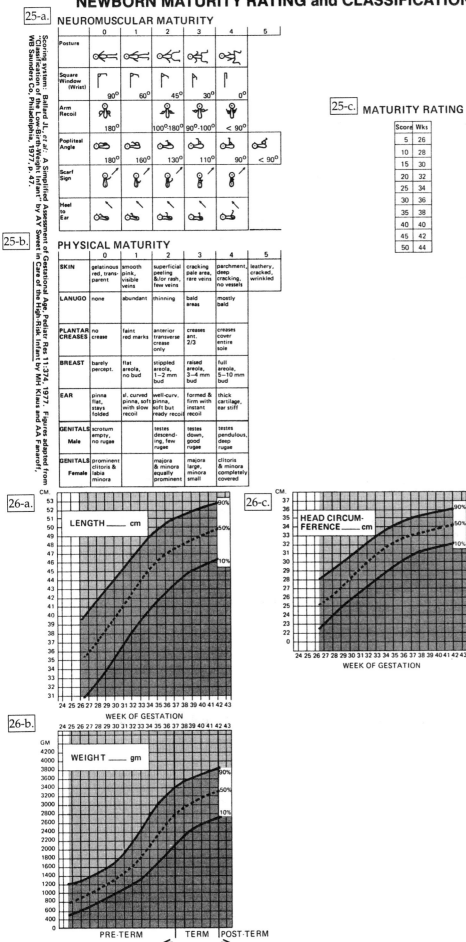

25-a. NEUROMUSCULAR MATURITY

25-b. PHYSICAL MATURITY

25-c. MATURITY RATING

Score	Wks
5	26
10	28
15	30
20	32
25	34
30	36
35	38
40	40
45	42
50	44

Scoring system: Ballard JL, et al: A Simplified Assessment of Gestational Age. Pediatr Res 11:374, 1977. Figures adapted from "Classification of the Low-Birth-Weight Infant" by AY Sweet in Care of the High-Risk Infant by MH Klaus and AA Fanaroff, WB Saunders Co, Philadelphia, 1977, p. 47.

26-a. LENGTH _____ cm

26-b. WEIGHT _____ gm

26-c. HEAD CIRCUMFERENCE _____ cm

Multiple Choice

Situation: *During the physical examination of a 21 year old female, the following was observed: dry skin, lanugo hair pattern, stunted growth pattern, and a weight loss of 85% the expected height.*

29. Which one of the following is a risk factor that requires further assessment?
    A. Birth weight
    B. Family statutes
    C. Perceptual disturbance
    D. Skin care

30. Which one of the following is an estimate of frame size?
    A. Head diameter
    B. Elbow breadth
    C. Hip circumference
    D. Trunk measurement

31. A formula used to assess nutritional status and total body fat is the:
    A. BMI.
    B. CAD.
    C. PIH.
    D. SMR.

32. A waist to hip circumference ratio over 0.9 in men and 0.8 in women suggests a/an:
    A. healthy nutritional status.
    B. decreased amount of body fat.
    C. increased risk for disease.
    D. overuse of steroids.

33. A correlation exists between the triceps skinfold thickness and the body's:
    A. electrolyte balance.
    B. fat content.
    C. hair distribution.
    D. muscle mass.

34. Which cultural group tends to weigh less at birth than white North american infants?
    A. American Indian
    B. Black American
    C. Native Hawaiian
    D. Native Norwegian

35. Which cultural group tends to have higher maturity scores of term infants at birth?
    A. Asian Americans
    B. Black Americans
    C. Native Americans
    D. White Americans

36. When would a sitting height measurement be indicated in a child?
    A. After the newborn is assessed as AGA.
    B. At every clinic or office visit.
    C. If the body proportions appear unusual.
    D. When growth is within normal range.

37. What condition may exist when a child's arm span is greater than his or her height?
    A. Acromegaly
    B. Diabetes
    C. Marfan syndrome
    D. Turner syndrome

Situation: *An adolescent hispanic child has a shorter height measurement than children of other cultural groups. She asks her health care provider if she is normal.*

38. You should know that her height is a/an:
    A. condition requiring further tests.
    B. expected finding for her cultural group.
    C. indication of disease or disorder.
    D. pathologic finding that needs treatment.

39. The averaging of a girl's stage of pubic hair and breast development or a boy's stage of pubic hair and genital development is a/an:
    A. BMR.
    B. FHT.
    C. HTN.
    D. SMR.

Situation: *Ms. G. is being seen for a routine physical examination. Her weight is 85% of the expected weight for her age and stature. She states that her figure has remained the same for the past few years. When asked questions about her nutrition, she replies that she needs to get back to work.*

40. The examiner should evaluate the possibility that Ms. G. has:
    A. achondroplasia.
    B. anorexia nervosa.
    C. growth hormone deficit.
    D. hypopituitary dwarfism.

Matching

	Findings	Terms
_____	41. Excess caloric intake causing excess fat	A. Achondroplasia
_____	42. Weight loss from disease process	B. Acromegaly
_____	43. Facial prominence in middle age from excess growth hormone	C. Cachexia
_____	44. Moon face from steroid therapy	D. Cushingoid face
_____	45. Fat resulting from metabolic or endocrine disorder	E. Endogenous obesity
_____	46. Dwarfism with endochondral ossification	F. Exogenous obesity
_____	47. Abnormality of sex chromosomes	G. Turner's syndrome

NURSING CONSIDERATIONS

Completion

48. In the space provided, describe at least one technique or guideline you would want to teach patients about doing their own daily weight measurements.

_____

_____

_____

Situation: *Mr. D. is an overweight person seeking assistance to correct his eating habits. He states that he eats because of his work stress. His triceps skinfold measurement is greater than 15 mm. Mr. D.'s weight, height and frame shows that he has more than a 30% gain over his ideal weight. He states that he does not routinely exercise. He also reports missing his wife who recently divorced him.*

49. State a nursing diagnosis appropriate to Mr. D.'s situation.

_____

50. List at least one subjective data and one objective finding from the above scenario that are defining characteristics.

A. *Subjective:* _____

_____

B. *Objective:* _____

_____

Chapter 5

Skin, Hair, and Nails

LEARNING OBJECTIVES

After (1) reading the textbook chapter, pages 131–183, (2) studying nursing considerations for Skin, Hair, and Nails in Part II of this workbook, and (3) completing the following questions, students should be able to:

ANATOMY AND PHYSIOLOGY

1. Recognize anatomy of the skin, hair, and nails.
2. Describe physiology of the skin, hair, and nails.
3. Identify age and condition variations in the skin, hair, and nails.

HISTORY

4. Select patient information relevant to the present problem data of a skin, hair, and nail history.
5. Gather personal and social history data pertinent to a skin, hair, and nail assessment.
6. Collect past medical and family data relevant to a skin, hair, and nail history.
7. Compile age and condition data relevant to a skin, hair, and nail history.

EXAMINATION

8. Identify appropriate equipment for a skin, hair, and nail assessment.

Indicate appropriate techniques for a skin, hair, and nail assessment by:

9. inspection;
10. palpation;
11. measurements; and
12. transillumination.

FINDINGS

13. Recognize expected findings from a skin, hair, and nail examination.
14. Assess variations of minor consequence in skin, hair, and nail findings.
15. Evaluate expected age and condition variations in skin, hair, and nail findings.
16. Assess potential disorders and abnormalities of the skin, hair, and nails.
17. Appraise age and condition variations suggesting disorders or abnormalities of the skin, hair, and nails.

NURSING CONSIDERATIONS

18. Evaluate cultural factors pertinent to a skin, hair, and nail assessment.
19. Apply critical thinking towards analyzing nursing considerations during a skin, hair, and nail examination.
20. Formulate appropriate nursing diagnoses after completing a skin, hair, and nail assessment.

STUDY FOCUS

The hair, skin, and nails are the "face" ever present to the world. As you complete these exercises, focus on their structures and underlying physiology. The astute observations of the examiner during the history and physical examination will give many insights to the overall well being of the patient.

ANATOMY AND PHYSIOLOGY

Completion

1. Label the diagram of the nail by placing the correct term beside each letter.

   A. _____

   B. _____

   C. _____

   D. _____

   E. _____

2. What is the process by which the skin accomplishes each of the following functions?

   A. Retards fluid loss by _____

   B. Repairs surface wounds by _____

   C. Contributes to blood pressure regulation by _____

   D. Regulates body temperature by _____

Matching

	Characteristics	*Life Cycle*
_____	3. Dry skin and hair	A. Adolescents
_____	4. Odorless sweat	B. Infants
_____	5. Oily skin	C. Older adults
_____	6. Sweaty hands and feet	D. Pregnant women

TRUE or Corrected Statement

_____ 7. Sweat glands, hair, and nails are all formed from invaginations of epidermis into dermis.

_____ 8. Middle Easterners have less apocrine gland enlargement and excretion during adolescence.

_____ 9. Ridges on the finger nails are typical in pregnant women.

_____ 10. Closely packed dead squamous cells that provide waterproofing keratin are found in the stratum corneum.

HISTORY

Completion

11. State at least one reason why each of the following data should be assessed as part of a patient's personal and social history.

    A. Exposure to occupational hazards: _____

    _____

    B. Hair care: _____

    _____

    C. Medications: _____

    _____

    D. Nail care: _____

    _____

    E. Recent stress: _____

    _____

    F. Sun exposure: _____

    _____

12. Describe at least two pieces of data pertinent to the history of a child.

    A. _____

    B. _____

13. Describe at least two pieces of data pertinent to the history of an older adult.

    A. _____

    B. _____

EXAMINATION

Completion

14. Describe how you would perform each of the following assessments.

A. Determination of size of lesion: _____

_____

B. Nuances of color, elevation, and border: _____

_____

C. Presence of fungal infections: _____

_____

D. Elevation or depression of lesion: _____

_____

E. Skin temperature: _____

_____

F. Turgor and mobility: _____

_____

TRUE or Corrected Statement

_____ 15. Tangential lighting is best used for inspecting skin <u>color</u>.

_____ 16. Skin temperature is best assessed with the <u>dorsal surfaces</u> of the examiner's hands.

_____ 17. Fluorescing lesions are seen best with a <u>transilluminator</u>.

_____ 18. Examination of the skin is performed by inspection and <u>percussion</u>.

_____ 19. Centimeter rulers should be <u>inflexible and opaque</u>.

FINDINGS

TRUE or Corrected Statement

_____ 20. <u>Bulging veins</u> is an "ABCD" characteristic of malignant melanoma.

_____ 21. <u>American Indians</u> have the lowest incidence of nevi.

_____ 22. A dark band is a normal finding on the nails of <u>mongoloid infants</u>.

_____ 23. <u>Anonychia</u> may occur as a congenital condition.

Matching

	Characteristics	*Nevus*
_____	24. Dome shaped, raised	A. Compound
_____	25. Flat or slightly elevated	B. Hairy
_____	26. Indistinct border	C. Halo
_____	27. May be present at birth	D. Intradermal
_____	28. Sharp, oval or circular	E. Junction

Conditions

_____ 29. Albinism, vitiligo
_____ 30.. Cardiac or pulmonary problem
_____ 31. Fever, polycythemia
_____ 32. Liver disease
_____ 33. Pituitary, adrenal disorder

Cutaneous Color

A. Blue
B. Brown
C. Red
D. White
E. Yellow

Examples

_____ 34. Acne
_____ 35. Blister
_____ 36. Freckle
_____ 37. Psoriasis
_____ 38. Wart

Lesions

A. Bulla
B. Macule
C. Papule
D. Plaque
E. Pustule

Findings

_____ 39. Circumscribed, silvery scales
_____ 40. Erythematous, pruritic rash
_____ 41. Hot, red, tender, indurated
_____ 42. Pustules with inflammation
_____ 43. Soft, mobile, elevated lesion
_____ 44. Swollen or purulent on dermatome

Abnormalities

A. Cellulitis
B. Drug eruption
C. Folliculitis skin
D. Herpes zoster
E. Psoriasis
F. Squamous cell CA

Completion

45. Under each picture and short description write the name of the lesion and state whether its type is primary or secondary.

a.

Irregular macular patches

A. Name _____
   Lesion Type _____

b.

Heaped-up keratinized cells

B. Name _____
   Lesion Type _____

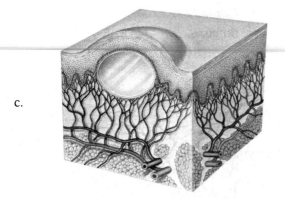

c.

Elevated and filled with fluid

C. Name _____

    Lesion Type _____

d.

Excessive collagen

D. Name _____

    Lesion Type _____

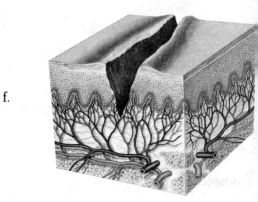

e.

1 to 2 cm in diameter

E. Name _____

    Lesion Type _____

f.

Break from epidermis to dermis

F. Name _____

    Lesion Type _____

Multiple Choice

Situation: *You are examining a four-week-old black neonate. You notice a large blue-black spot on the buttock. The mother states that the infant was born with it.*

46. You would know that this finding:
    - A. is an expected finding.
    - B. may indicate child abuse.
    - C. relates to birth trauma.
    - D. suggests a congenital defect.

47. Breast feeding, hemolytic disease, and bleeding are risk factors associated with:
    - A. acrocyanosis within 24 hours of life.
    - B. colic during the newborn period.
    - C. hyperbilirubinemia in the newborn.
    - D. sleep apnea in the infant or toddler.

48. A skin lesion that may be associated with neurofibromatosis or pulmonary stenosis is:
    A. cafe au lait spots.
    B. epidermal verrucous nevi.
    C. Faun tail nevus.
    D. port wine limb stain.

49. When does hair on the extremities typically become darker and more coarse?
    A. At birth
    B. After menopause
    C. During pregnancy
    D. With puberty

50. An increase in pigmentation and the development of linea nigra may occur:
    A. at birth.
    B. after menopause.
    C. during pregnancy.
    D. with puberty.

51. Which decubitus ulcer stage indicates damage through the epidermis and dermis?
    A. Stage I
    B. Stage II
    C. Stage III
    D. Stage IV

52. Which lesion is an expected finding on the skin of healthy older adults?
    A. Acne vulgaris
    B. Cherry angiomas
    C. Miliaria
    D. Trichotillomania

53. A superficial area of hyperkeratosis is called a:
    A. callus.
    B. clavus.
    C. corporis.
    D. corn.

54. Painful, itching and burning "shingles" is a viral infection resulting from:
    A. drug eruptions.
    B. herpes simplex.
    C. herpes zoster.
    D. pityriasis rosea.

55. Which malignant tumor arises in the epithelium and occurs most commonly in sun–exposed areas?
    A. Basal cell carcinoma
    B. Kaposi sarcoma
    C. Malignant melanoma
    D. Squamous cell carcinoma

56. Which condition occurs with rubeola?
    A. Kopliks spots
    B. Mongolian spots
    C. Solar keratosis
    D. Strawberry hemangioma

NURSING CONSIDERATIONS

57. Which defining characteristic is most likely to be associated with impaired skin integrity related to pressure from immobilization?
    A. Alert patient
    B. Coccyx lesion
    C. Hypertension
    D. Self care

58. An example of a subjective defining characteristic is:
    A. blister.
    B. cyanosis.
    C. erythema.
    D. itching.

59. Inadequate secondary defenses is an example of a:
    A. history notation.
    B. nursing definition.
    C. nursing diagnosis.
    D. related factor.

Situation: Mr. W. has a left hand rash that appeared about a month ago. His fungal examination and skin cultures are negative. Mr. W. states that his rash itches badly. His left hand is more red than his right hand. Mr. W. has been doing yard work for the last few weeks.

60. Which nursing diagnosis is most appropriate?
    A. Activity intolerance: high risk
    B. Coping: ineffective individual
    C. Impaired skin integrity: high risk
    D. Tissue perfusion: impaired

Chapter 6

Lymphatic System

LEARNING OBJECTIVES

After (1) reading the textbook chapter, pages 184–208, (2) studying nursing considerations for the Lymphatic System in Part II of this workbook, and (3) completing the following questions, students should be able to:

ANATOMY AND PHYSIOLOGY

1. Recognize anatomy of the lymphatic system.
2. Describe physiology of the lymphatic system.
3. Identify age and condition variations in the lymphatic system.

HISTORY

4. Select patient information relevant to the present problem data of a lymphatic history.
5. Gather personal and social history data pertinent to a lymphatic assessment.
6. Collect past medical and family data relevant to a lymphatic history.
7. Compile age and condition data relevant to a lymphatic history.

EXAMINATION

8. Identify appropriate equipment for lymphatic assessment.

Indicate appropriate techniques for lymphatic assessment by:

9. Inspection;
10. Palpation; and
11. Measurement and transillumination of any masses.

FINDINGS

12. Recognize expected findings from a lymphatic examination.
13. Assess variations of minor consequence in lymphatic findings.
14. Evaluate expected age and condition variations in lymphatic findings.
15. Assess potential disorders and abnormalities of the lymphatic system.
16. Appraise age and condition variations suggesting disorders or abnormalities of the lymphatic system.

NURSING CONSIDERATIONS

17. Evaluate cultural factors pertinent to lymphatic assessment.
18. Apply critical thinking towards analyzing nursing considerations during lymphatic assessment.
19. Formulate appropriate nursing diagnoses after completing a lymphatic system examination.

STUDY FOCUS

The lymphatic system and the immunologic system are interrelated. This chapter reviews the structure and purpose of lymphatic drainage. You will learn the importance of evaluating superficial lymph nodes to assess health and potential disorders.

LEARNING ACTIVITIES

ANATOMY AND PHYSIOLOGY

Completion

1. Draw the following groups of nodes onto the diagram. Clearly label these nodes by placing each term to the side of the diagram with a line to the nodes.

   Bronchial
   Iliac
   Inguinal
   Mediastinal
   Mesentery
   Preaortic
   Trachel

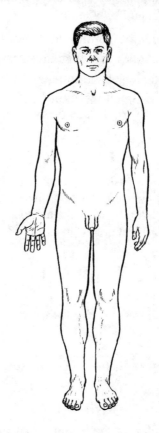

2. List five functions or activities of the lymphatic system.
   A. _____
   B. _____
   C. _____
   D. _____
   E. _____

Matching

Descriptions	*Terms*
_____ 3. Arise from precursor cells	A. Lymph nodes
_____ 4. Has white and red pulp	B. Lymphocytes
_____ 5. In connective tissue, muscles, and body cavities	C. Spleen
_____ 6. In superior mediastinum	D. Thymus
_____ 7. Organized as follicles and crypts	E. Tonsils

TRUE or Corrected Statement

_____ 8. Cells that line the lymph node sinuses perform the specific function of phagocytosis.

_____ 9. Lymph ducts merge into the venous system at the vena cava.

_____ 10. The internal structure that is largest in proportion to the rest of the body at birth and reaches its greatest absolute weight at puberty is the spleen.

_____ 11. Lymph nodes of older adults are more likely to be smooth.

HISTORY

Completion

Situation: During a history and physical, Ms. R states that she has recently experienced sore, bleeding gums.

12. Describe three types of data you would collect concerning Ms. R's complaints.

A. _____

_____

B. _____

_____

C. _____

_____

13. List at least four conditions a family member might have that would be pertinent to a lymphatic history.

A. _____

B. _____

C. _____

D. _____

EXAMINATION

Multiple Choice

14. Which item is used for assessing lymph nodes?
    A. Centimeter ruler
    B. Skin calipers
    C. Tanner scale
    D. Wood's lamp

15. Which technique is used to detect edema, erythema, and lesions?
    A. Goniometer readings
    B. Inspection of areas
    C. Microscopic viewing
    D. Palpation of nodes

16. Which statement is correct concerning the mnemonics "PALS" for assessing and documenting an enlarged lymph node?
    A. A= All associated nodes
    B. L= Length of erythema
    C. P = Palpable fatty tissue
    D. S = Swelling of extremities

17. To palpate lymph node clusters, the hand should probe without pressing hard and be moved in a:
    A. circular fashion.
    B. downward motion.
    C. random manner.
    D. sideways maneuver.

Matching

	Six Step Order of Head Palpation	*Location*
_____	18. 1–Occipital nodes	A. At angle of mandible
_____	19. 2–Postauricular nodes	B. At base of skull
_____	20. 3–Preauricular nodes	C. Between angle and mandible tip
_____	21. 4–Tonsillar nodes	D. In front of ears
_____	22. 5–Submaxillary nodes	E. Midline, behind mandibletip
_____	23. 6–Submental nodes	F. Over mastoid process

FINDINGS

TRUE or Corrected Statement

_____ 24. Lymph nodes are <u>large and stationary</u> in a healthy person.

_____ 25. Tenderness is almost always indicative of <u>cancer</u>.

_____ 26. Transillumination is done to distinguish nodes <u>from cysts</u>.

_____ 27. The <u>harder and more discrete</u> the node, the more likely it is to be malignant.

_____ 28. Normal lymph nodes of children under age two may be <u>oval shaped</u>.

_____ 29. <u>Thyroglossal duct cysts</u> may cause nasopharynx obstruction and sleep apnea.

_____ 30. <u>Branchial cleft cyst</u> may simulate lymph node enlargement.

_____ 31. <u>Cervical adenitis</u> will obscure the angle of the jaw.

_____ 32. <u>Acute lymphangitis</u> is the inflammation of one or more lymphatic vessels

_____ 33. With <u>AIDS</u> you may find red streaks or fine lines leading toward an extremity.

_____ 34. <u>Hodgkin disease</u> is a malignant lymphomas occurring in young people of all races.

_____ 35. Palatal petechiae is a common finding with <u>elephantiasis</u>.

_____ 36. Splenomegaly and hepatomegaly are frequent findings with <u>Epstein–Barr virus mononucleosis</u>.

_____ 37. Enlarged anterior cervical and submandibular nodes may occur with <u>Herpes simplex</u>.

_____ 38. Initial symptoms of <u>lymphoma</u> include lymphadenopathy, fatigue, and weight loss.

_____ 39. Acquired <u>lymphedema</u> results from regional node duct trauma.

_____ 40. <u>Milroy disease</u> may cause a disruption of lymphatic circulation in the legs.

NURSING CONSIDERATIONS

Multiple Choice

Situation: You are examining an 18-month-old child for an upper respiratory infection. The mother states that this is her baby's first "cold." The child's history reflects a healthy family with no known risk factors for infection.

41. Which of the following findings would require additional assessment before you would be ready to write a nursing diagnosis?
    A. Discrete axillary nodes
    B. Enlarged spleen
    C. Runny and red nose
    D. Small cervical nodes

Situation: A physical examination of a 75-year-old woman's forearm revealed acute lymphangitis and axillary lymph node enlargement. You trace the fine lines that are on the extremity. Before completing this patient's nursing diagnosis, you further evaluate her inflammation.

42. The most probable site of infection for this patient would be her:
    A. breast.
    B. hand.
    C. neck.
    D. shoulder.

43. When addressing nursing considerations, a patient's biographic data should be reported as part of the:
    A. defining characteristics.
    B. diagnostic evaluation.
    C. health history.
    D. physical examination.

44. Traumatized tissue is a risk factor most associated with infection and:
    A. adequate secondary defense.
    B. decreased physical capability.
    C. inadequate primary defenses.
    D. nutritional concerns.

45. Which of the following represents an objective finding pertinent to the nursing diagnosis of activity intolerance related to fatigue from an infectious process?
    A. Describes tired feelings
    B. Expresses lack of energy
    C. Misses school days
    D. Wants to sleep

Modified Matching

Characteristic	Data
_____ 46. Describes tiredness	"S" = SUBJECTIVE
_____ 47. Decreased libido	"O" = OBJECTIVE
_____ 48. Lethargy	
_____ 49. Listlessness	
_____ 50. Sits frequently	

Chapter 7

Head and Neck

LEARNING OBJECTIVES

After (1) reading the textbook chapter, pages 209–234, (2) studying nursing considerations for the Head and Neck in Part II of this workbook, and (3) completing the following questions, students should be able to:

ANATOMY AND PHYSIOLOGY

1. Recognize anatomy of the head and neck.
2. Describe physiology of the head and neck.
3. Identify age and condition variations in the head and neck.

HISTORY

4. Select patient information relevant to the present problem data of a head and neck history.
5. Gather personal and social history data pertinent to a head and neck assessment.
6. Collect past medical and family data relevant to a head and neck history.
7. Compile age and condition data relevant to a head and neck history.

EXAMINATION

8. Identify appropriate equipment for a head and neck assessment.

Indicate appropriate techniques for a head and neck assessment by:

9. Inspection;
10. Palpation;
11. Auscultation; and
12. Measurement and transillumination.

FINDINGS

13. Recognize expected findings from a head and neck examination.
14. Assess variations of minor consequence in head and neck findings.
15. Evaluate expected age and condition variations in head and neck findings.
16. Assess potential disorders and abnormalities of the head and neck.
17. Appraise age and condition variations suggesting disorders or abnormalities of the head and neck.

NURSING CONSIDERATIONS

18. Evaluate cultural factors pertinent to a head and neck assessment.
19. Apply critical thinking towards analyzing nursing considerations during a head and neck examination.
20. Formulate appropriate nursing diagnoses after completing a head and neck assessment.

STUDY FOCUS

There are many structures that compose the head and neck. The major structures, including bones, muscles, tendons and blood vessels are reviewed. Pertinent head and neck information gathered in a history may involve several different systems. Study the types of data, such as nutritional information and past surgeries, that are important to the history. The equipment, examination steps and findings from a head and neck examination vary, depending on the age and condition of the patient. Use the following questions to test your knowledge base.

LEARNING ACTIVITIES

ANATOMY AND PHYSIOLOGY

Completion

1. Use the following terms to label the diagram of the skull. Place the correct term in the lettered answer space. Use each term once.

Condyloid process
Coronal suture
External acoustic meatus
Frontal bone
Lambdoidal suture
Mandible
Mastoid process
Maxilla
Occipital bone
Parietal bone
Sphenoid bone
Squamous suture
Temporal bone
Zygomatic arch
Zygomatic bone

A. _____	F. _____	K. _____
B. _____	G. _____	L. _____
C. _____	H. _____	M. _____
D. _____	I. _____	N. _____
E. _____	J. _____	O. _____

2. Use the following terms to label the diagram of the neck. Place the correct term in the lettered answer space. Use each term once.

Carotid sinus
Common carotid
  artery
Cricoid cartilage
External carotid
  artery
External jugular
  vein
Hyoid bone
Internal carotid
  artery
Jugular vein
Lymph node
Pyramidal lobe
Thyroid cartilage
Thyroid gland
Trachea

A. _____   F. _____   K. _____
B. _____   G. _____   L. _____
C. _____   H. _____   M. _____
D. _____   I. _____
E. _____   J. _____

3. Complete the following statements by placing the answers in the blanks.
   A. Ossification of the sutures begins around age _____.
   B. The posterior fontanel closes around age _____.
   C. The anterior fontanel usually closes by age _____.

Multiple Choice
4. The skull is composed of:
   A. 2 bones.
   B. 7 bones.
   C. 10 bones.
   D. 21 bones.

5. The relationship of muscles and adjacent bones in the head serve as anatomic landmarks since they form:
   A. indentations.
   B. right angles.
   C. triangles.
   D. vascularities.

6. Which structure is located in the upper ring of the tracheal cartilage?
   A. Angle of Louis
   B. Condyloid process
   C. Cricoid cartilage
   D. Hyoid sinuses

7. The nose and thyroid cartilage enlarge in the male during:
   A. adolescence.
   B. early childhood.
   C. infancy.
   D. late adulthood.

8. When should you expect to see a slight enlargement of the thyroid gland because of hyperplasia and increased vascularity?
   A. After menopause
   B. At puberty
   C. During pregnancy
   D. In childhood

HISTORY

Situation: You are taking the history of a 23-year-old woman who has persistent, recurring headaches. She states that she never had headaches until about 18 months ago.

9. Which of the following risk factors is most important to assess?
   A. Aspirin ingestion
   B. Contraception used
   C. Exercise pattern
   D. Job stress

Situation: Ms. L. noticed a nodular tenderness in her throat. Her family doctor suggested that she have additional tests for a potential thyroid problem.

10. What data is most pertinent to Ms. L.'s history?
    A. Change in menstrual flow
    B. Evidence of polydactyly
    C. Increase in lacrimation
    D. Presence of nevi

TRUE or Corrected Statement

_____ 11. One general consideration in a history is the patient's consumption of milk.

_____ 12. Problem related data addressed in a history includes <u>visual prodromal event</u>.

_____ 13. Data pertinent to a medical history includes surgery for <u>koilonychia</u>.

_____ 14. Data on family history that should be addressed is incidence of <u>gonad dysfunction</u>.

_____ 15. An example of age related information is <u>encephalocele</u>.

Completion

Situation: *Mr. T arrived in emergency from his construction job site. His helmet was off when he hit his head on a protruding pipe. His co–worker insisted that Mr. T seek health care, even though he seemed all right. Mr. T had drunk several beers the night before and stated that he wanted to go back to work so he wouldn't lose his job.*

16. List four items of general data about Mr. T that need to be obtained.

A. _____
B. _____
C. _____
D. _____

EXAMINATION

17. List four types of equipment you would assemble before performing a head and neck examination, and explain their uses.

Equipment	Uses
A. _____	A. _____
B. _____	B. _____
C. _____	C. _____
D. _____	D. _____

18. Describe at least two characteristics that can be assessed by inspection of the head and face of an adult.

A. _____
B. _____

19. Delineate how you would assess a temporal bruit.

_____
_____

20. Explain either the frontal or the posterior method for palpation of the thyroid.

_____

_____

_____

_____

21. Describe how you would transilluminate the skull of a newborn.

_____

_____

_____

FINDINGS

Multiple Choice

22. An indentation or depression of the skull may indicate a:
    A. degenerative change.
    B. hypertensive incident.
    C. skull fracture.
    D. vascular anomaly.

23. A salivary gland with an infection or ductal stone is likely to cause a/an:
    A. discrete nodule.
    B. increase in salivation.
    C. enlarged, tender gland.
    D. jaw lock or tic.

24. Neck webbing, excessive posterior cervical skin, and a short neck are signs associated with:
    A. Asian races.
    B. chromosomal anomalies.
    C. excessive exercise.
    D. malnutrition.

25. What is the significance of a visible, moving thyroid gland in a patient who is swallowing?
    A. Cricoid cartilage has been injured
    B. Movement is a sign of cancer
    C. The thyroid gland is enlarged
    D. Visibility is a usual finding

Situation: Examination of a neonate 10 hours after birth revealed generalized subcutaneous scalp edema. The parents verbalize concern.

26. Which of the following is the best response to give these concerned parents?
    A. A collection of blood is under the scalp causing swelling.
    B. Newborn head swelling is due to birth trauma.
    C. Such swelling is common and should gradually disappear.
    D. Unusual head contours are sometimes seen in newborns.

27. Preterm infants often have:
    A. broad nose bridges.
    B. long, narrow heads.
    C. low set ears.
    D. wide, fat necks.

28. The presence of a nodular thyroid is a normal finding in:
    A. adolescents.
    B. infants.
    C. older adults.
    D. pregnant women.

29. A patient with left mouth and eye lid sagging is likely to have:
    A. facial nerve paralysis.
    B. facial muscle weakness.
    C. peripheral trigeminal nerve irritation.
    D. ocular motor nerve degeneration.

30. A "moon" shaped face, erythematous skin, and hirsutism are typical characteristics of:
    A. craniofacial dysostosis.
    B. Cushing syndrome.
    C. Graves disease.
    D. systemic lupus.

Completion

31. Give three reasons why you may find a patient's head tilted to the left side.
    A. _____
    B. _____
    C. _____

32. Contrast at least four system or structural differences between hyperthyroidism and hypothyroidism.

A. _____

_____

B. _____

_____

C. _____

_____

D. _____

_____

Matching

Headache Type

	Characteristic
_____ 33. Classic migraine	A. Alcohol consumption
_____ 34. Cluster	B. Constricting pain
_____ 35. Common	C. Fluid retention
_____ 36. Hypertensive	D. Occipital location
_____ 37. Muscular tension	E. Older onset
_____ 38. Temporal arteris	F. Prodromal scotoma

Description

	Conditions
_____ 39. Adult onset of hypothyroidism	A. Brachial cleft cyst
_____ 40. Autoimmune thyroid	B. Graves disease
_____ 41. Cystic neck mass; disorder	C. Myxedema
_____ 42. Injury during birth	D. Torticollis
_____ 43. Mass near sternocleidomastoid; embryologic remnant	E. Thyroglossal duct cyst fetal remnant

NURSING CONSIDERATIONS

Multiple Choice

44. Which finding is most likely to be related to a nursing diagnosis of sleep pattern disturbance related to increased metabolic rate and restlessness?
    A. Blood pressure of 130/70
    B. Decreased body temperature
    C. Elevated T_3 and T_4
    D. Ten pound weight gain

45. Where in the health history would you document a patient's nervousness and neck discomfort?
    A. Chief complaint
    B. Present problem
    C. Past Medical
    D. Personal and Social

46. Which nursing diagnosis is appropriate to a patient with negative feelings about self?
    A. Body image disturbance
    B. Individual coping problem
    C. Negative self concept
    D. Self image problem

Modified Matching

	Characteristic	*Data*
_____	47. Appetite loss	"S" = Subjective data
_____	48. Has tenderness	"O" = Objective data
_____	49. Heat sensitivity	
_____	50. Is perspiring	

Chapter 8

Eyes

LEARNING OBJECTIVES

After (1) reading the textbook chapter, pages 235–268, (2) studying nursing considerations for the Eyes in Part II of this workbook, and (3) completing the following questions, students should be able to:

ANATOMY AND PHYSIOLOGY

1. Recognize anatomy of the eyes.
2. Describe physiology of the eyes.
3. Identify age and condition variations in the eyes.

HISTORY

4. Select patient information relevant to the present problem data of an eye history.
5. Gather personal and social history data pertinent to an eye assessment.
6. Collect past medical and family data relevant to an eye history.
7. Compile age and condition data relevant to an eye history.

EXAMINATION

8. Identify appropriate equipment for an eye assessment.
Indicate appropriate techniques for an eye assessment by:
9. Inspection;
10. Visual testing;
11. Muscle testing; and
12. Ophthalmoscopic examination.

FINDINGS

13. Recognize expected findings from an external eye examination.
14. Assess expected findings from an ophthalmoscopic examination.
15. Evaluate expected age and condition variations in eye findings.
16. Assess potential disorders and abnormalities of the eyes.
17. Appraise age and condition variations suggesting disorders or abnormalities of the eyes.

NURSING CONSIDERATIONS

18. Evaluate cultural factors pertinent to an eye assessment.
19. Apply critical thinking towards analyzing nursing considerations during an eye examination.
20. Formulate appropriate nursing diagnoses after completing an eye assessment.

STUDY FOCUS

The sensory organ for seeing involves an intricate relationship between external and internal eye structures. An eye examination includes the evaluation of sight, as well as the assessment of conditions that indicate underlying pathology. While answering the following questions, consider methods for obtaining history data and physical findings. Review the connection between normal anatomy and physiology, and the subjective and objective data that you will collect. Study potential risk factors and common abnormalities related to the eyes.

LEARNING ACTIVITIES

ANATOMY AND PHYSIOLOGY

Completion

1. Use the following terms to label the diagram of the cross section of the eye. Place the correct term in the lettered answer space. Use each term once.

Anterior chamber
Choroid
Ciliary body
Cornea
Iris muscle
Lens

Macular area
Optic nerve
Retina
Sclera
Vitreous body

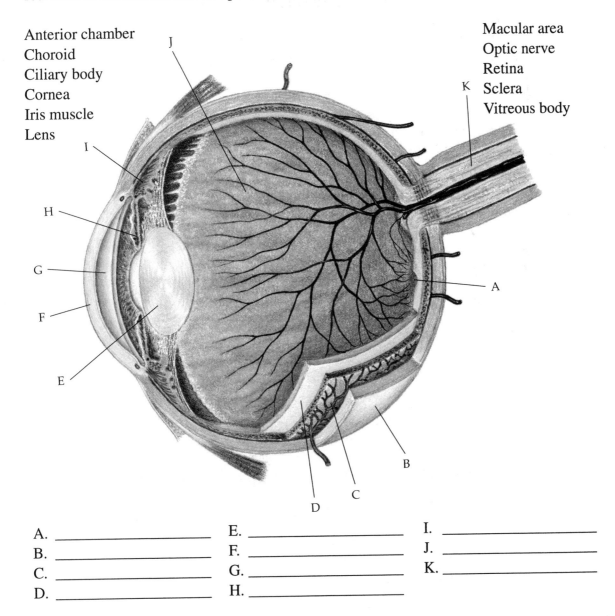

A. _____   E. _____   I. _____
B. _____   F. _____   J. _____
C. _____   G. _____   K. _____
D. _____   H. _____

2. Write at least one function of each of the following structures in the space provided.

A. Eyelids: _____

B. Conjunctiva: _____

C. Lacrimal glands: _____

D. Sclera: _____

E. Cornea: _____

F. Iris: _____

G. Lens: _____

H. Retina: _____

Matching

	Characteristics	*Structure*
_____	3. Biconvex and transparent	A. Cornea
_____	4. Color of the eye	B. Iris
_____	5. Senses pain	C. Lens
_____	6. Sensory network	D. Retina
_____	7. White of the eye	E. Sclera

Multiple Choice

8. The thin membrane that covers the anterior eye surface is the:
   A. choroid coat.
   B. conjunctiva.
   C. cornea.
   D. lacrimal region.

9. What eye structure is continuous with the sclera?
   A. Choroid coat
   B. Conjunctiva
   C. Cornea
   D. Lacrimal region

10. The infant gains voluntary control of the eye muscles around what age?
    A. 2 months
    B. 4 months
    C. 6 months
    D. 8 months

11. Until 6 years of age, eyeballs are less spherical than those of adults, which accounts for why children have:
   A. ciliary muscle weakness.
   B. fiber compression.
   C. lense rigidity.
   D. myopic acuity.

12. The eyes have corneal edema and thickening, Krukenberg spindles, and an increase of lysozyme:
   A. at birth.
   B. after menopause.
   C. during pregnancy.
   D. throughout puberty.

HISTORY

13. Which one of the following would be assessed as part of the family history?
   A. Contact lenses
   B. Eye color
   C. Pupil size
   D. Retinoblastoma

14. Current ptosis of the lids that result in vision obstruction is an example of data belonging in the:
   A. family history.
   B. past medical history.
   C. present problem.
   D. social history.

Completion

15. Name six areas of information that you would seek to understand a chief complaint of "I don't see well."
   A. _____
   B. _____
   C. _____
   D. _____
   E. _____
   F. _____

16. Explain in the space provided why the academic performance would be important data to the eye history of a child.
   _____
   _____

EXAMINATION

17. List at least three items that would be needed for an eye assessment.
    A. _____
    B. _____
    C. _____

18. Name three important principles to be applied when you use the Snellen eye test for visual acuity.
    A. _____
    B. _____
    C. _____

19. Describe how you would estimate an adult patient's peripheral vision.
    _____
    _____
    _____

20. List in order the external eye structures that should be examined. To the right of each structure, write at least one reason for examining it.

Structure	*Reason*
A. _____	A. _____
	_____
B. _____	B. _____
	_____
C. _____	C. _____
	_____
D. _____	D. _____
	_____
E. _____	E. _____
	_____
F. _____	F. _____
	_____

21. Explain why you should shine a tangential light at the limbus before instilling mydriatics.
    _____
    _____

22. Explain why an ophthalmoscope has a red and a black lens setting.
    _____
    _____
    _____

23. State how you would test visual acuity in a 15–month–old child.

_____

_____

FINDINGS

Multiple Choice

Situation: Ms. C. has vision that is not correctable to better than 20/200. There has been little change in her visual abilities for several years.

24. Ms. C. is considered to be:
    A. legally blind.
    B. mildly myopic.
    C. moderately hyperostic.
    D. unilaterally anisocoric.

25. Thyroid hypoactivity, allergies, and renal disease may cause which finding?
    A. Edema of orbital area
    B. Scleral brown spots
    C. Strabismus and tearing
    D. Weak ciliary muscle

26. When the lower eye lid is turned away from the eye, the condition is called:
    A. ectropion.
    B. entropion.
    C. exophthalmus.
    D. paresis.

27. A cobblestone appearance of the conjunctiva is most likely related to:
    A. cancer.
    B. cataracts.
    C. hyperlipidemia.
    D. infection.

28. Lid lag may indicate:
    A. coma.
    B. diabetes.
    C. hyperthyroidism.
    D. pregnancy.

29. Which structure is usually yellow to creamy pink?
    A. Conjunctivae
    B. Disc
    C. Iris
    D. Lens

30. Which cultural group is more likely to have pseudostrabismus?
    A. Alaskan Eskimos
    B. East Indians
    C. Native Americans
    D. Scandinavians

Situation: Examination of a 43-year-old female revealed bilateral exophthalmos. Her condition is exaggerated by retraction of the upper lid and sclera exposure.

31. This finding is suggestive of:
    A. carcinoma.
    B. Graves disease.
    C. myxedema.
    D. torticollis.

32. Which finding is of primary concern when examining the eyes of a 32-year-old male with juvenile onset diabetes?
    A. Brown dots with pink periphery edges
    B. Creamy disc area with distinct borders
    C. Pink drusen bodies that float freely
    D. Yellow spots with poorly defined margins

33. A condition that is associated with anoxia and the development of new vessels is:
    A. diabetic retinopathy.
    B. homonymous hemianopia.
    C. pregnancy-induced hypertension.
    D. retinal fibroplasia.

Matching

	Associated Factors	*Abnormality*
_____	34. Acute angle glaucoma	A. Adie pupil
_____	35. Congenital finding in 20% of those healthy	B. Anisocoria
		C. Argyll Robertson pupil
_____	36. Diminished tendon reflexes often occur	D. Mydriasis
_____	37. Increased intracranial pressure	E. Oval pupil
_____	38. Neurosyphilis or midbrain lesion	

Characteristics	Condition
_____ 39. Blurred vision and ocular pain occur	A. Band keratopathy
_____ 40. Common with Crohn's disease	B. Cataracts
_____ 41. Congenital malignant tumor	C. Corneal ulcer
_____ 42. Increased risk when contact	D. Episcleritis
lenses are worn	E. Exophthalmos
_____ 43. More common in Blacks and	F. Glaucoma
Mediterranean descent	G. Retinitis pigmentosa
_____ 44. Most common with hyperparathyroidism	H. Retinoblastoma
_____ 45. Night blindness occurs	
_____ 46. Occurs in most individuals after age 65	

NURSING CONSIDERATIONS

Multiple Choice

47. Which nursing diagnosis relates to an individual who experiences a change in interpretation of stimuli by sight receptors?
    A. Altered kinesthetic function
    B. Diversional activity deficit
    C. Impaired tactile/visual interaction
    D. Visual sensory/perceptual alteration

48. Which of the following is a subjective defining characteristic?
    A. Headache
    B. Inflammation
    C. Squinting
    D. Tearing

Completion

Situation: Ms. S, age 79, expresses concern about her decreasing sight. Her ophthalmologist recently told her that she needs cataract surgery. She verbalizes confusion about her diagnosis and treatment. Ms. S. states that: "I wish that I didn't have glaucoma. My sister had glaucoma."

49. Compose an appropriate nursing diagnosis related to Ms. S.

_____

50. List at least two related factors that may be associated with the nursing diagnosis "Sensory/Perceptual Alteration: Visual."

    A. _____

    B. _____

Chapter 9

Ears, Nose, and Throat

STUDY FOCUS

The ears and nose, like the eyes, are sensory organs. Head orifices, including the mouth and throat, have several functions. Hearing, smelling, breathing, eating and even walking are related to the health of these passageways. Complete the following questions while asking yourself what conditions influence the functioning of the ears, nose, and throat.

LEARNING ACTIVITIES

ANATOMY AND PHYSIOLOGY

Completion

1. Use the following terms to label the diagram of the nose and nasopharynx. Place the correct term in the lettered answer space. Use each term once.

Cribriform plate
Eustachian tube
Frontal sinus
Hard palate
Inferior turbinate

Middle turbinate
Soft palate
Sphenoidal sinus
Superior turbinate

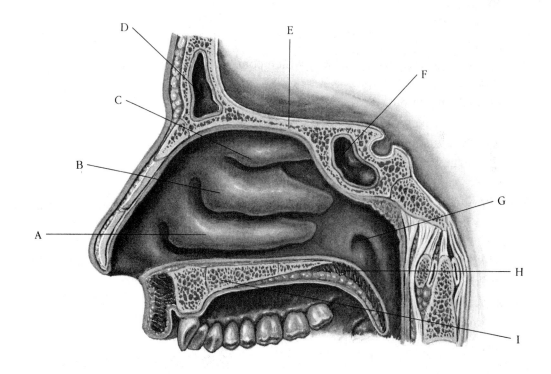

A. _____

B. _____

C. _____

D. _____

E. _____

F. _____

G. _____

H. _____

I. _____

2. Describe the process of hearing.

_____
_____
_____
_____
_____

Multiple Choice

3. Ossicles and the tympanic membrane are housed in the:
   A. footplate.
   B. middle ear.
   C. sebaceous glands.
   D. vestibular branch.

4. Equalizing atmospheric pressure when yawning, sneezing or swallowing is accomplished by what ear structure?
   A. Eustachian tube
   B. Pars faccida
   C. Short process
   D. Triangular fossa

5. Oriental individuals are likely to have which condition more frequently than other cultural groups?
   A. Colds and flu symptoms
   B. Inner ear balance problems
   C. Nonerupted wisdom teeth
   D. Overly large frenulum

Situation: Sally has recently experienced voice hoarseness and a persistent cough. Her voice has a periodic cracking sound. You know that these symptoms are an expected finding for Sally.

6. It is likely that Sally is:
   A. a toddler.
   B. approaching puberty.
   C. experiencing menopause.
   D. pregnant.

Situation: You are examining a patient who has a short external canal that curves upward. The eustachian tube is short and wide.

7. This patient is probably a:
   A. college student
   B. middle school student
   C. newborn or toddler
   D. retired person

Completion

8. Why do pregnant women experience nasal stuffiness, fullness in the ears, and impaired hearing?

   _____
   _____

9. Give four reasons that older adults experience hearing loss.
   A. _____
   B. _____
   C. _____
   D. _____

HISTORY

10. Compose at least one question that should be asked as part of the medical history for an ear, nose, and throat assessment.

    _____
    _____

11. Describe the significance of a family history of hereditary renal disease to an ear, nose, and throat history.

    _____
    _____
    _____

12. Describe infant behaviors that may suggest a hearing loss.

    _____
    _____
    _____

EXAMINATION

Matching

	Patient's Anatomic Factors	*Technique*
_____	13. Head toward opposite shoulder	A. Otoscopic exam
_____	14. Light against supraorbital rims	B. Rinne test
_____	15. One ear obstructed from hearing	C. Transillumination
_____	16. Tuning fork on mastoid bone	D. Weber test
_____	17. Tuning fork on midline vertex	E. Whisper test

Completion

18. Describe two ways to prevent ear pain from an otoscopic examination.

    A. _____

    _____

    B. _____

    _____

19. Describe the technique for palpating the tongue and gums.

    _____

    _____

TRUE or Corrected Statement

_____ 20. In the presence of otitis externa, tympanic membrane perforation, or myringotomy tubes you should <u>clean the inner ear with soap</u>.

_____ 21. The <u>Rinne test</u> is used to evaluate lateralization of sound.

_____ 22. An otoscopic and oral examination in a child should usually be performed <u>at the beginning of the assessment</u>.

FINDINGS

Completion

23. Explain how you would determine whether redness in a child's tympanic membrane was from crying or infection.

    _____

    _____

24. Describe the expected nasal muscosal color and the usual mucosal color of an allergic nose.

    _____

    _____

25. Describe the expected findings for each of the following assessments.
    A. Proper closure of teeth: _____

    _____

    B. Stensons duct: _____

    _____

    C. Gums: _____
    D. Tongue: _____
    E. Hard palate: _____

    _____

    F. Tonsils: _____

    _____

Matching

	Characteristics		Prominent Group
_____	26. Dry cerumen more common	A.	Blacks
_____	27. Fissured tongue is usual	B.	Elderly
_____	28. Has tendency for small teeth	C.	Orientals
_____	29. Higher incidence of lip pits	D.	Whites
_____	30. More likely to have otosclerosis	E.	Women

TRUE or Corrected Statement

_____ 31. A newborn whose serum bilirubin is greater than 20 mg/100 ml risks later tooth decay.

_____ 32. Bulging of the tympanic membrane without mobility is most often associated with impacted cerumen in the canal.

_____ 33. Nasal turbinates that are grayish or pinkish with a boggy, swollen appearance suggests cocaine use.

_____ 34. Pharyngitis is considered a medical emergency.

_____ 35. Tonsils that appear pushed backward or forward with a displaced uvula suggests a peritonsillar abscess.

_____ 36. Presbycusis is an expected finding with advancing age.

_____ 37. A functional assessment helps to evaluate adequate nutrition.

Matching

	Findings		Terms
_____	38. Dry mouth; systemic disease	A.	Labyrinthitis
_____	39. Ear fullness; tinnitus	B.	Meinere disease
_____	40. Fever, headache and nasal discharge	C.	Sinusitis
_____	41. Soft palate petechial marks	D.	Tonsillitis
_____	42. Vertigo; nystagmus	E.	Xerostomia

Multiple Choice

43. Ear canal itching, pain with chewing, and watery or purulent discharge may indicate that the patient has:
    A. bacterial otitis media
    B. infected sinuses
    C. secretory otitis media
    D. swimmer's ear

44. Which condition is caused by either a congenital defect or chronic infection and results in a blue or red tympanic membrane and growth of keratinizing squamous epithelium?
    A. Cauliflower ear
    B. Cholesteatoma
    C. Cochleatitis
    D. Craniofacial fissures

45. Which of the following is a hereditary condition that occurs more frequently in women and results in fixed stapes from irregular labyrinthine ossification?
    A. Darwin tubercle
    B. Eustachian engorgement
    C. Kiesselbach plexus
    D. Otosclerosis

46. Chronic sniffling, nasal congestion, nosebleeds, mucosal scabs and septum perforation are signs of:
    A. chronic allergies.
    B. cocaine abuse.
    C. fungal exposure.
    D. legionnaire's disease.

47. An obstruction in airflow or a failure of the central nervous system to stimulate the respiratory effort to breath may result in:
    A. choanal atresia.
    B. cleft palate.
    C. presbycusis.
    D. sleep apnea.

NURSING CONSIDERATIONS

48. Tinnitus would be considered a/an:
    A. nursing diagnosis.
    B. objective observation.
    C. related factor
    D. subjective finding.

49. A subjective finding of vertigo and an objective finding of motor incoordination would be recorded as part of the:
    A. defining characteristics.
    B. diagnostic procedures.
    C. nursing diagnosis.
    D. related factors.

Completion

50. List at least five factors that may be related to a nursing diagnosis of "Sensory/Perceptual Alteration: Auditory."
    A. _____
    B. _____
    C. _____
    D. _____
    E. _____

Chapter 10

Chest and Lungs

LEARNING OBJECTIVES

After (1) reading the textbook chapter, pages 314–366, (2) studying nursing considerations for the Chest and Lungs in Part II of this workbook, and (3) completing the following questions, students should be able to:

ANATOMY AND PHYSIOLOGY

1. Recognize anatomy of the chest and lungs.
2. Describe physiology of the chest and lungs.
3. Identify age and condition variations in the chest and lungs.

HISTORY

4. Select patient information relevant to the present problem data of a chest and lung history.
5. Gather personal and social history data pertinent to a chest and lung assessment.
6. Collect past medical and family data relevant to a chest and lung history.
7. Compile age and condition data relevant to a chest and lung history.

EXAMINATION

8. Identify appropriate equipment for a chest and lung assessment.

Indicate appropriate techniques for a chest and lung assessment by:

9. Inspection;
10. Palpation;
11. Percussion; and
12. Auscultation and measurement

FINDINGS

13. Recognize expected findings from a chest and lung examination.
14. Assess variations of minor consequence in chest and lung findings.
15. Evaluate expected age and condition variations in chest and lung findings.
16. Assess potential disorders and abnormalities of the chest and lungs.
17. Appraise age and condition variations suggesting disorders or abnormalities of the chest and lungs.

NURSING CONSIDERATIONS

18. Evaluate cultural factors pertinent to a chest and lung assessment.
19. Apply critical thinking towards analyzing nursing considerations during a chest and lung examination.
20. Formulate appropriate nursing diagnoses after completing a chest and lung assessment.

STUDY FOCUS

While finishing this workbook chapter, study the structure of the thorax and the function of the respiratory system. Interrelate history data with expected findings and common abnormalities of the chest and lungs. Respiratory findings are often associated with other systemic conditions. Remember to look, listen and feel in a thorough and integrated manner.

LEARNING ACTIVITIES

ANATOMY AND PHYSIOLOGY

TRUE or Corrected Statement

_____ 1. The apex of the lung is <u>even with the second rib</u>.

_____ 2. On deep inspiration, the lower lung borders descent to <u>T8</u>.

_____ 3. The <u>manubrium</u> contains all the thoracic viscera except the lungs.

_____ 4. The trachea is anatomically below the <u>larynx</u>.

_____ 5. The <u>bronchi</u> transports air and removes noxious materials.

_____ 6. The terminal bronchioles subdivide to respiratory <u>bronchioles</u>, each of which is associated with one acinus.

_____ 7. Changes in oxygen and carbon dioxide levels stimulate chemoreceptors in the <u>parietal and visceral pleurae</u>.

_____ 8. The lung begins forming at <u>14 weeks</u> gestation.

_____ 9. Increased oxygen in the arterial blood of a newborn causes <u>hyper–inflation of the lungs</u>.

_____ 10. Dry mucous membranes and increased residual volume are usual findings <u>during adolescence</u>.

Completion

11. Opposite each structure describe its role or function.

Structure	Function
A. Chemoreceptors in medulla oblongata	A. _____ _____ _____ _____
B. Chemoreceptors in carotid body	B. _____ _____ _____ _____
C. Medulla oblongata	C. _____ _____
D. Pons	D. _____ _____
E. Placenta	E. _____ _____

12. How is adequate ventilation maintained in a pregnant woman despite the decrease in lung length and rise in diaphragm?

_____

_____

_____

_____

13. Why are older people dyspneic on heavy exertion and predisposed to respiratory infections?

_____

_____

_____

_____

HISTORY

14. Explain why smoking of family members is pertinent to a chest and lung history.

_____

_____

_____

15. Explain why weight change is important data on the chest and lung history of older adults.

_____

_____

_____

Multiple Choice

16. Which risk factor is most important to evaluate in a young person having severe, acute chest pain?
    A. Anorexia nervosa
    B. Cocaine use
    C. Pregnancy potential
    D. Rheumatic fever

Situation: Your are conducting a chest and lung history on Mr. L. He states that he cannot get rid of his cold. His skin color is good. Mr. L. is a nonsmoker.

17. Which one of the following is most important to Mr. L.'s history?
    A. Allergy tests and treatment plans
    B. Expectations for treatment and care
    C. Experiences with difficult breathing
    D. Previous sports injuries and rehabilitation

Situation: Ms. R. has had asthma for several years. She has an extensive medical chart.

18. Which data are most important to Ms. R.'s past medical history?
    A. Number of pillows usually used
    B. Onset and duration of current problem
    C. Skin test results done for fungus
    D. Typical use of tobacco products

19. A risk factor for a potential respiratory disability is:
    A. age from birth to young adulthood.
    B. family history of hypertension.
    C. female gender with "XX" chromosomes.
    D. previous respiratory infections.

EXAMINATION

20. Which of the following equipment is useful during a chest and lung examination?
    A. Calipers
    B. Eyeliner
    C. Goniometer
    D. Sextant

21. When should you inspect the patient's chest?
    A. After the patient begins to cough
    B. While the patient breathes naturally
    C. While the patient holds his or her breath
    D. With your palm on the patient's chest

22. During percussion, the patient holds his or her arms in front in order to:
    A. expose maximum lung area.
    B. make the ribs protrude.
    C. prevent attacks of coughing.
    D. recognize thudlike sounds.

23. Which equipment transmits high pitched sound when auscultating the lungs?
    A. Bell device
    B. Doppler transducer
    C. Stethoscope diaphragm
    D. Ultrasonic microphone

24. The correct procedure for lung auscultation is to listen:
    A. during expiration.
    B. during inspiration.
    C. for 15–30 seconds.
    D. through inspiration and expiration.

25. When you auscultate the lungs first at the lung base and then at the apex, you can best distinguish:
    A. different coughing sounds.
    B. pneumonia from asthma.
    C. rales from rhonchi.
    D. wheezing from emphysemic rubs.

26. The Hamman sign can best be heard when the patient is:
    A. in a supine position.
    B. lying on the left side.
    C. sitting completely upright.
    D. with the head elevated 30 degrees.

27. When you note cyanosis, pursed lips, clubbing of fingers, and nasal flaring, you are using the technique of:
    A. auscultation.
    B. inspection.
    C. palpation.
    D. percussion.

Completion

28. Describe the technique for evaluating thoracic expansion during respirations.
    _____
    _____
    _____

29. Summarize the main principles that guide the steps for measurement of diaphragmatic excursion.
    _____
    _____
    _____
    _____

FINDINGS

30. Name seven findings that indicate healthy lungs.
    A. _____
    B. _____
    C. _____
    D. _____
    E. _____
    F. _____
    G. _____

31. An infant received a 1-minute Apgar score of 9 with 1 point subtracted for acrocyanosis. What is the most likely reason for the acrocyanosis?

_____

_____

Matching

Findings

_____ 32. Air in subcutaneous tissue
_____ 33. Increased dyspnea when upright
_____ 34. Prominent sternal protrusion
_____ 35. Stridor and chest wall caving
_____ 36. Tactile fremitus over bronchi

Interpretation

A. Crepitus
B. Expected finding
C. Pigeon chest
D. Platypnea
E. Retractions

Completion

37. Use the following terms to label the diagram of the chest. Match the sound with the area where it is most likely to be heard. Use each sound term once. Place the correct term in the lettered answer space.

Bronchial: coarse, loud
Rhonchi: coarse, low-pitched
Bronchovesicular: combination sounds
Crackles: fine crackling, high-pitched

Rub: scratchy, high-pitched
Tracheal: coarse, loud
Vesicular: high-pitched, breezy
Wheeze: whistling, high-pitched rhonchus

A. _____ D. _____ G. _____
B. _____ E. _____ H. _____
C. _____ F. _____

Matching

Findings

_____ 38. Continuous, deep rumbling during expiration

_____ 39. Discrete, discontinuous, millisecond sounds

_____ 40. High pitched sounds over trachea with long expiration

_____ 41. Low pitched, dry grating sounds throughout breathing cycle

_____ 42. Low pitched, soft sound over normal lung tissue

Interpretation

A. Bronchial sounds
B. Crackles
C. Friction rub
D. Rhonchi
E. Vesicular sounds

Findings

_____ 43. Air trapped in expiration

_____ 44. Booming percussion note

_____ 45. Dullness to percussion

_____ 46. Muted breath sounds

_____ 47. Round chest in 3-year old

Interpretation

A. Atelectasis
B. Cystic fibrosis
C. Emphysema
D. Pneumonia
E. Pneumothorax

NURSING CONSIDERATIONS

Multiple Choice

Situation: Mr. M. has COPD. His arterial blood gases show lower O_2 and higher CO_2 levels than his usual results. Mr. M. is alert and willing to talk. You are conducting his health history and are evaluating nursing considerations appropriate to Mr. M.'s situation.

48. It would be most appropriate to:
   A. conduct short sessions with rest periods.
   B. copy Mr. M.'s previous history from his chart.
   C. encourage Mr. M. to answer open–ended questions.
   D. use a standard form to collect Mr. M.'s data.

Situation: You are reviewing diagnostic results for a respiratory patient in preparation for analyzing special nursing considerations. Your patient is a minority to the dominant American citizen.

49. You should recall that race and weight influence:
   A. blood gas results.
   B. chest X–ray readings.
   C. hematology reports.
   D. lung function tests.

Situation: Your patient is having difficulty maintaining airway patency. You are composing a nursing diagnosis of <u>ineffective airway clearance</u>.

50. Which one of the following is a correct completion of your nursing diagnosis?
    INEFFECTIVE AIRWAY CLEARANCE:
    A. Associated with complaints of fatigue.
    B. Occurring with dyspnea and rhonchi.
    C. Patient verbalizes inability to cough.
    D. Related to the effects of anesthesia.

Chapter 11

Heart and Blood Vessels

LEARNING OBJECTIVES

After (1) reading the textbook chapter, pages 367-443, (2) studying nursing considerations for the Heart and Blood Vessels in Part II of this workbook, and (3) completing the following questions, students should be able to:

ANATOMY AND PHYSIOLOGY

1. Recognize anatomy of the heart and blood vessels.
2. Describe physiology of the heart and blood vessels.
3. Identify age and condition variations in the heart and blood vessels.

HISTORY

4. Select patient information relevant to the present problem data of a heart and blood vessel history.
5. Gather personal and social history data pertinent to a heart and blood vessel assessment.
6. Collect past medical and family data relevant to a heart and blood vessel history.
7. Compile age and condition data relevant to a heart and blood vessel history.

EXAMINATION

8. Identify appropriate equipment for a heart and blood vessel assessment.

Indicate appropriate techniques for a heart and blood vessel assessment by:

9. Inspection;
10. Palpation;
11. Percussion; and
12. Auscultation and measurement.

FINDINGS

13. Recognize expected findings from a heart and blood vessel examination.
14. Assess variations of minor consequence in heart and blood vessel findings.
15. Evaluate expected age and condition variations in heart and blood vessel findings.
16. Assess potential disorders and abnormalities of the heart and blood vessels.
17. Appraise age and condition variations suggesting disorders or abnormalities of the heart and blood vessels.

NURSING CONSIDERATIONS

18. Evaluate cultural factors pertinent to a heart and blood vessel assessment.
19. Apply critical thinking towards analyzing nursing considerations during a heart and blood vessel examination.
20. Formulate appropriate nursing diagnoses after completing a heart and blood vessel assessment.

STUDY FOCUS

Cardiovascular health involves a complicated network of structures and an intricate set of physiologic functions. Family history and life style habits are particularly important to the well being of a human heart and its supporting vessels. Examination techniques and subsequent interpretations are outlined in the following exercises. Concentrate on the interrelationship of anatomy, physiology, history, examination protocols and findings while you review nursing considerations.

LEARNING ACTIVITIES

ANATOMY AND PHYSIOLOGY

Completion

1. Where is the heart usually located in relation to the following?
   A. Mediastinum: _____
   B. Diaphragm: _____
   C. Lungs: _____
   D. Sternum: _____
   E. Tall slender person: _____
   F. Short stocky person: _____

2. Describe the position of the following parts and surface areas of the heart in relation to each other.
   A. Right ventricle: _____
   B. Left ventricle: _____
   C. Right atrium: _____
   D. Left atrium: _____

3. Where in the heart is each of the following located?
   A. Tricuspid valve: _____
   B. Mitral valve: _____
   C. Pulmonic valve: _____
   D. Aortic valve: _____

Matching

	Description	Term
_____	4. Atrial blood fills relaxed ventricles	A. Afterload
_____	5. Closure of mitral and tricuspid valves	B. Dextrocardia
_____	6. Force challenging ventricle muscles	C. Diastole
_____	7. Mirror image of usual heart position	D. Preload
_____	8. Pulmonic and aortic valves forced open	E. Systole

80

Completion

9. Place the correct term in the lettered answer space. (Optional: After completing this exercise, label other heart anatomy, such as the apex and ventricles. You could also draw and label chest structures directly onto the diagram, e.g., rib, spinal or respiratory structures surrounding the heart.

Aorta
Aortic valve
Inferior vena cava
Left common carotid artery
Left pulmonary artery
Left subclavian artery
Mitral valve

Pulmonic valve
Right common carotid artery
Right pulmonary artery
Right subclavian artery
Superior vena cava
Tricuspid valve

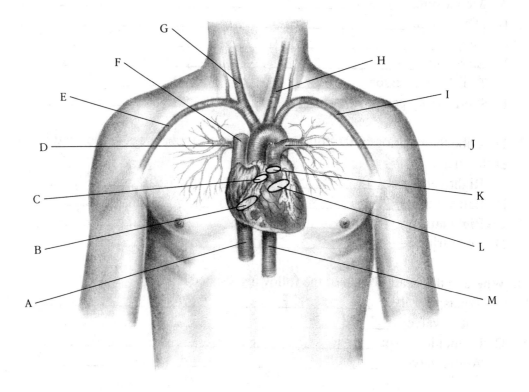

A. _____

B. _____

C. _____

D. _____

E. _____

F. _____

G. _____

H. _____

I. _____

J. _____

K. _____

L. _____

M. _____

10. Define the following five "S" heart sounds.

S1: _____

_____

S2: _____

S3: _____

S4: _____

_____

Split S2: _____

_____

_____

11. Explain the following three terms.

A. Depolarization: _____

_____

B. Repolarization: _____

_____

C. Stroke volume: _____

_____

12. Name five physiologic variables that affect pulses.

A. _____

B. _____

C. _____

D. _____

E. _____

Matching

Definitions

_____ 13. Atrial depolarization

_____ 14. Final phase of ventricular repolarization

_____ 15. Time from initial stimulation of atria
       to initial stimulation of ventricles

_____ 16. Ventricular depolarization

_____ 17. Ventricular repolarization

Terms (Place only letter(s) on line to indicate matching definition)

P wave

PR interval

QRS complex

T wave

U wave

Completion

18. How does the position of the heart in infants and children under age 7 differ from that of adults?

_____

_____

19. Why does blood pressure drop during early pregnancy?

_____

_____

_____

20. Name at least two changes in the following structures and system that are due to aging.
   A. Heart:
   1. _____

   _____

   2. _____

   _____

   B. Arteries:
   1. _____

   _____

   2. _____

   _____

   C. Conduction system:
   1. _____

   _____

   2. _____

   _____

HISTORY

21. Name at least five items of information that you would seek about a patient's chest pain.
   A. _____

   _____

   B. _____

   _____

   C. _____

   _____

   D. _____

   _____

   E. _____

   _____

Modified Matching

Chest Pain History

_____	22. Awakened with early morning pain
_____	23. Continues even if effort stopped
_____	24. Difficulty falling asleep
_____	25. Disappears when exertion ceased
_____	26. Previous incident of trauma
_____	27. Related to indigestion
_____	28. Related to emotional effort
_____	29. Relief with antacids
_____	30. Relief with heat and aspirin

Pain Source

AP = Angina pectoris
MS = Musculoskeletal
GI = Gastrointestinal

Matching

History Data

_____	31. Cardiac disability
_____	32. Feeding exhaustion
_____	33. Hemoptysis
_____	34. Nosebleeds
_____	35. Proteinuria
_____	36. Varicosities

Most Likely Group

A. Children
B. Infants
C. Irish or German descent
D. Older adults
E. Pregnant women
F. Young men

EXAMINATION

TRUE or Corrected Statement

_____ 37. A goniometer is used to assess the heart and blood vessels.

_____ 38. An apical pulse is usually visible in the third right intercostal space.

_____ 39. To estimate heart size by percussion, you should begin tapping at the midclavicular line.

_____ 40. Percussion is of limited value due to chest rigidity and heart conformity.

_____ 41. To hear diastolic heart sounds, you should ask patients to sit up and lean forward.

_____ 42. The bell of the stethoscope is more useful than the diaphragm for hearing protodiastolic gallops.

_____ 43. You should bilaterally palpate both carotid arteries at the same time.

_____ 44. A Trendelenburg test evaluates patency of deep veins.

_____ 45. To distinguish a murmur from respiration, briefly bend the baby's head down.

Completion

46. List four methods for facilitating auscultation of heart sounds.

A. _____

B. _____

C. _____

D. _____

47. How would you make it easy for yourself to asucultate an arterial bruit?

_____

_____

48. How would you measure a blood pressure in the leg, and what is the expected finding?

_____

_____

_____

FINDINGS

Multiple Choice

Situation: You are palpating over the base of a patient's heart. When you reach the second intercostal space, you palpate a rushing vibration.

49. This finding indicates a:

A. heave.

B. lift.

C. thrill.

D. thrust.

50. Which sound results from the closure of the semilunar valves?

A. S_1

B. S_2

C. S_3

D. S_4

Situation: You are auscultating a patient's heart and find a grade II murmur without radiation. The murmur has a medium pitch. The patient's chart has a previous notation about the murmur. You learn that this murmur is a non-problematic, common variation.

51. This patient is a/an:

A. elderly woman.

B. middle aged man.

C. pregnant woman.

D. school aged child.

52. Atherosclerosis, anemia, anxiety and exercise are associated most with which type of arterial pulse?
    A. Alternating pulse
    B. Bounding pulse
    C. Labile pulse
    D. Paradoxic pulse

53. Which one of the following murmurs results from valvular aortic stenosis?
    A. Aortic stenosis
    B. Carotid artery bruit
    C. Clavicular thrill
    D. Pulmonic regurgitation

Situation: Vascular assessment of a 42-year-old man with deep vein thrombosis revealed severe occlusion. You decide to check his capillary refill times.
54. Which of the following results is most likely?
    A. < 1 second
    B. < 2 seconds
    C. > 2 seconds
    D. No blanching

Situation: You suspect that Ms. D. has thrombosis. You have just dorsiflexed Ms. D.'s right foot. Ms. D. reports pain in her right calf.
55. This finding indicates a positive:
    A. Allis sign.
    B. Chadwick sign.
    C. Homan sign.
    D. Kehr sign.

56. Which age group is more likely to have liver enlargement before the lungs accumulate fluid due to heart failure?
    A. Adolescents
    B. Children
    C. Infants
    D. Older Adults

57. Severe hypertension accompanied by facial palsy is more common in:
    A. children.
    B. newborns.
    C. older adults.
    D. young adults.

Situation: Ms. T. has a blood pressure of 140/100. She is 34 weeks pregnant. Her pre-pregnant blood pressure was 108/68.

58. It is most likely that Ms. T. will:
    A. complete diagnostic tests related to diabetes.
    B. prepare for hospitalization for her PIH.
    C. receive nutritional instruction on salt restriction.
    D. return for re-evaluation in two weeks.

59. What disease process would you suspect if a patient reports a several week history of fever and shows clinical symptoms of congestive heart failure?
    A. Bacterial endocarditis
    B. Cardiac tamponade
    C. Infarction
    D. Myocarditis

60. What condition is most likely if a patient has an excessive accumulation of fluid or blood between the pericardium and heart?
    A. Bacterial endocarditis
    B. Cardiac tamponade
    C. Infarction
    D. Myocarditis

Matching

Findings

_____ 61. Diastolic rumble accentuated early and late in diastole, louder on inspiration.

_____ 62. Early diastolic murmur, high pitch, blowing

_____ 63. Low-frequency diastolic rumble, opening snap

_____ 64. Midsystolic murmur, medium pitch, coarse thrill

_____ 65. Murmur fills systole, medium pitch, coarse thrill

_____ 66. Systolic murmur, medium pitch, thrill, ejection click after S_1

Conditions

A. Aortic regurgitation
B. Aortic stenosis
C. Mitral stenosis
D. Pulmonic stenosis
E. Subaortic stenosis
F. Tricuspid stenosis

Description

_____ 67. ECG pattern is saw toothed

_____ 68. Excessive, regular heart beats

_____ 69. Irregular muscle wall spasms

Term

A. Atrial fibrillation
B. Atrial flutter
C. Atrial tachycardia

Description	Term
_____ 70. Conduction disrupted	A. Heart block
_____ 71. Electrical source in ventricles	B. Ventricular fibrillation
_____ 72. Complete loss of regular rhythm	C. Ventricular tachycardia

TRUE or Corrected Statement

_____ 73. Coarctation of the aorta is a combination of four cardiac defects.

_____ 74. Continuation of fetal circulation is situs inversus.

_____ 75. A thrill or bruit is often heard over a fistula.

_____ 76. Acute rheumatic fever is a systemic connective tissue disease.

_____ 77. Midsystolic ejection murmur is a typical finding with venous ulcers.

NURSING CONSIDERATIONS

Multiple Choice

Situation: You are reviewing patient clinic records in order to prepare for patient teaching that you will conduct. You determine that the same test has been planned for a patient with a suspected rhythm disturbance, a patient with a pacemaker, and another patient on anti-arrhythmic therapy.

78. You decide to conduct a small group session for these patients who will most likely have a/an:
    A. angiography.
    B. echocardiogram.
    C. holter monitor.
    D. stress test.

79. Which nursing diagnosis is most likely to be appropriate to the related factors of reduced stroke volume secondary to a congenital abnormality?
    A. Cardiac output, decreased
    B. Colonic function, impaired
    C. Fluid volume excess
    D. Peripheral–neurovascular dysfunction

80. Defining characteristics of guarding, grimacing, and moaning are:
    A. objective data.
    B. patient symptoms.
    C. related factors.
    D. subjective signs

LEARNING OBJECTIVES

After (1) reading the textbook chapter, pages 444–470, (2) studying nursing considerations for the Breasts and Axillae in part II of this workbook, and (3) completing the following questions, students should be able to:

ANATOMY AND PHYSIOLOGY

1. Recognize anatomy of the breasts and axillae.
2. Describe physiology of the breasts and axillae.
3. Identify age and condition variations in the breasts and axillae.

HISTORY

4. Select patient information relevant to the present problem data of a breast and axilla history.
5. Gather personal and social history data pertinent to a breast and axilla assessment.
6. Collect past medical and family data relevant to a breast and axilla history.
7. Compile age and condition data relevant to a breast and axilla history.

EXAMINATION

8. Identify appropriate equipment for a breast and axilla assessment.

Indicate appropriate techniques for a breast and axilla assessment by:

9. Inspection; and
10. Palpation with patient in different positions.

FINDINGS

11. Recognize expected findings from a breast and axilla examination.
12. Assess variations of minor consequence in breast and axilla findings.
13. Evaluate expected age and condition variations in breast and axilla findings.
14. Assess potential disorders and abnormalities of the breasts and axillae.
15. Appraise age and condition variations suggesting disorders or abnormalities of the breasts and axillae.

NURSING CONSIDERATIONS

16. Evaluate cultural factors pertinent to a breast and axilla assessment.
17. Apply critical thinking towards analyzing nursing considerations during a breast and axilla examination.
18. Formulate appropriate nursing diagnoses after completing a breast and axillae assessment.

STUDY FOCUS

An understanding of breast anatomy and physiology is needed so that a thorough examination can be conducted and patient education can be provided. Specific information relevant to a breast and axillae history is important to preventive care. Learn the sequential steps for performing a breast and axillae examination. In your mind, contrast findings that may or may not suggest pathology.

LEARNING ACTIVITIES

ANATOMY AND PHYSIOLOGY

TRUE or Corrected Statement

_____ 1. The glandular tissue of the female breast is organized into lobes, <u>lobules</u>, ducts, and acini cells.

_____ 2. The subcutaneous and retromammary fat provide <u>support</u> to the female breast.

_____ 3. Vascular supply to the breast is primarily through branches of the internal mammary and lateral <u>thoracic</u> arteries.

_____ 4. The greatest amount of glandular tissue in the female breast is in the <u>tail of Spence</u>.

_____ 5. <u>Pectoralis minor muscle</u> contraction causes erection of nipples and lactiferous ducts to empty.

_____ 6. Superficial lymphatics drain the <u>mammary lobules</u>.

_____ 7. The pectoral nodes are located along the lower border of the <u>pectoralis major</u> inside the lateral axillary fold.

_____ 8. Central lymph nodes are high in the <u>axilla</u> close to the ribs.

_____ 9. Colostrum is a product of increased <u>squamous</u> secretory activity.

_____ 10. Colostrum changes to high–protein transitional milk between the <u>third and sixth</u> days after delivery.

_____ 11. The average interval from the appearance of breast buds (stage II) to menarche is <u>3 months</u>.

_____ 12. During pregnancy, the production of luteal and placental hormones cause a <u>hardening of glandular tissue</u>.

_____ 13. Small, flat and loose nipples are most common in <u>premature infants</u>.

_____ 14. <u>After menopause</u>, glandular tissue is replaced by fat deposits in the breasts.

Completion

15. Draw the following structures onto the breast diagram. Clearly label these structures by placing each term to the side of the diagram with a line to the structure.

Alveolus
Clavicle
Lactiferous duct
Lactiferous sinus
Nipple pore
Pectoralis major muscle
Ribs
Suspensory ligaments

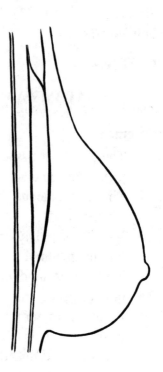

HISTORY

Situation: Ms. A., age 38, has come to the clinic because of nipple discharge. You are now interviewing her about her present problem. Thus far you have recorded this information: Patient has noticed watery yellow drainage from left nipple for past 2 months. No lump or discomfort. Left nipple is slightly retracted. No recent injury to breast. Takes no medications except Demulin. LMP = 12/10-12/26.

16. List at least two types of questions you will ask Ms. A as part of her history and state whether these data are part of the present problem, medical, family, age, or condition history.

A. _____

_____

B. _____

_____

Matching

	Description		History Section
_____	17. Age at menarche		A. Family history
_____	18. Breast cancer in sister		B. Past medical history
_____	19. Nipple discharge		C. Present problem
_____	20. Self examination habits		D. Personal history

Multiple Choice

21. Which risk factor may be associated with both breast cancer and benign breast disease?
    A. Early menopause
    B. Late menarche
    C. High income
    D. Low parity

22. Use of caffeine and alcohol is part of the:
    A. family history.
    B. past medical history.
    C. present problem.
    D. personal/social history.

EXAMINATION

Situation: You are preparing to examine Ms. E.'s breasts. She states that she has recently developed a nipple discharge on her left breast.

23. You will most likely need:
    A. a culture swab.
    B. a glass slide.
    C. formaldehyde.
    D. a pH strip.

Situation: You are helping a patient learn breast self examination techniques. Your patient, Ms. G., is 41 years old and states that she never checks her own breasts. Ms. G. has one child. She has had no previous breast problems.

24. Which one of the following should be recommended to Ms. G.?
    A. Conduct breast examinations two weeks after menses
    B. Have an initial mammogram by age 50
    C. Obtain professional examinations every 6 months
    D. Stand before a mirror during breast self examinations

Completion

25. Name seven types of data about the breasts you can obtain by inspection.

A. _____

B. _____

C. _____

D. _____

E. _____

F. _____

G. _____

26. Explain at least one reason that inspection of the breasts should continue with the woman in each of the following positions.

Position	*Reason*
A. Seated with arms overhead	A. _____ _____ _____
B. Seated with hands pressed against hips or palms pressed together	B. _____ _____ _____ _____
C. Seated leaning forward from waist.	C. _____ _____ _____

27. Name six important principles that guide the technique of breast palpation.

A. _____

B. _____

C. _____

D. _____

E. _____

F. _____

28. Describe the five steps for palpation of axillary nodes.

A. _____

B. _____

C. _____

D. _____

E. _____

FINDINGS

29. Retractions and dimpling caused by fibrotic tissue contraction is associated with:
    A. carcinoma.
    B. fibroids.
    C. lactation.
    D. nulliparity.

Situation: You are comparing the records of three patients. One patient is without venous patterns on her breasts. One patient has bilaterally visible patterns, and the other patient has noticeable venous patterns only on one breast.

30. Which patient needs additional assessment for possible breast pathology?
    A. The patient with bilateral patterns
    B. The patient without venous patterns
    C. The patient with unilateral patterns
    D. The two patients with venous patterns

31. A finding of nontender, nonsuppurative peppering of Montgomery tubercles is a:
    A. lymphatic infection.
    B. normal variation.
    C. pregnancy symptom.
    D. skin disease.

32. Supernumerary nipples are more common in which group of women?
    A. Blacks
    B. Eskimos
    C. Orientals
    D. Scandinavians

33. Most malignancies occur in the:
    A. muscles and nearby tendons.
    B. rib and xiphoid areas.
    C. tissue outside this region.
    D. upper outer breast quadrant.

Situation: Ms. O. has cyclical breast changes. She has noticed that these changes are less pronounced about a week after her menses start. Her last menstrual period was about three weeks ago. After taking Ms. O.'s history, you proceed with her examination.

34. Which of these findings would be typical for Ms. O.'s breasts?
    A. Asymmetry and dimpling
    B. Inverted cracked nipples
    C. Single solid mass
    D. Tenderness and nodularity

Situation: You are a nurse in a clinic when a women in her third trimester of pregnancy asks you about the drainage from her nipples. Her nipples are symmetric without redness.

35. Which response is most appropriate?
    A. Colostrum secretion is normal in the last trimester.
    B. Cultures should be done to rule out infection.
    C. Drainage indicates cancer and treatment is needed.
    D. Milk production indicates that delivery is eminent.

Matching

	Finding	*Most Likely Group*
_____	36. Inverted crusted nipple	A. Lactating women
_____	37. Firm disk of glandular tissue	B. Men
_____	38. Mastitis	C. Newborns
_____	39. Palpable inframammary ridge	D. Older women
_____	40. Witch's milk	E. Pregnant women

TRUE or Corrected Statement

_____ 41. Fibroadenoma is a non–cyclic, asymptomatic, benign breast tumor in young women.

_____ 42. Papillomatosis is a firm irregular mass resulting from local injury.

_____ 43. Fibrocystic disease is a surface manifestation of underlying ductal carcinoma.

_____ 44. Lactation resulting from certain medications or prolactin–secreting tumors is gynecomastia.

_____ 45. Blocked subareolar ducts during menopause is called mammary duct ectasia.

NURSING CONSIDERATIONS

Completion

46. State a nursing diagnosis for an individual who is having adaptive behavior problems related to unrealistic expectations concerning breast reconstruction following her mastectomy.

_____

Modified Matching

	Patient Following Mastectomy	*Defining Characteristic*
_____	47. Arm over left chest	**S** = Subjective
_____	48. Avoids looking at chest	**O** = Objective
_____	49. Negative self concept	
_____	50. Verbalizes shame	

Chapter 13

Abdomen

LEARNING OBJECTIVES

After (1) reading the textbook chapter, pages 471-529, (2) studying nursing considerations for the Abdomen in Part II of this workbook, and (3) completing the following questions, students should be able to:

ANATOMY AND PHYSIOLOGY

1. Recognize anatomy of the abdomen.
2. Describe physiology of the abdomen.
3. Identify age and condition variations in the abdomen.

HISTORY

4. Select patient information relevant to the present problem data of an abdominal history.
5. Gather personal and social history data pertinent to an abdominal assessment.
6. Collect past medical and family data relevant to an abdominal history.
7. Compile age and condition data relevant to an abdominal history.

EXAMINATION

8. Identify appropriate equipment for an abdominal assessment.

Indicate appropriate techniques for an abdominal assessment by:

9. Inspection;
10. Auscultation;
11. Percussion; and
12. Palpation.

FINDINGS

13. Recognize expected findings from an abdominal examination.
14. Assess variations of minor consequence in abdominal findings.
15. Evaluate expected age and condition variations in abdominal findings.
16. Assess potential disorders and abnormalities of the abdomen.
17. Appraise age and condition variations suggesting disorders or abnormalities of the abdomen.

NURSING CONSIDERATIONS

18. Evaluate cultural factors pertinent to an abdominal assessment.
19. Apply critical thinking towards analyzing nursing considerations during an abdominal examination.
20. Formulate appropriate nursing diagnoses after completing an abdominal assessment.

STUDY FOCUS

Several vital organs are housed in the abdominal cavity. Critical thinking skills should be used throughout an abdominal examination for interpreting the many findings associated with the abdominal organs and structures. Data from the history must be addressed systematically and thoroughly, in order to identify interrelationships between the many abdominal organs. Anatomic regions and landmarks are used to locate, record, and decipher findings.

LEARNING ACTIVITIES

ANATOMY AND PHYSIOLOGY

Completion

1. Draw the following structures onto the diagram. Clearly label these structures by placing each term to the side of the diagram with a line to the structure.

   Appendix
   Gallbladder
   Large intestine
   Liver
   Pancreas
   Small intestine
   Spleen

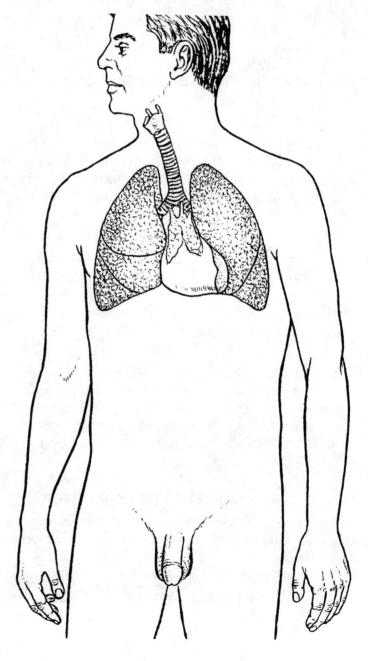

2. The kidneys lie behind some of the structures that you just drew. Place One X to indicate the location of the right kidney and another X to indicate the location of the left kidney.

Write the quadrant and region associated with the following structures. (The "Appendix" is completed as a sample.)

QUADRANT	STRUCTURE	REGION
RLQ	3. Appendix	R. inguinal
	4. Cecum	
	5. Duodenum	
	6. Left kidney	
	7. Left ureter	
	8. Right kidney	
	9. Right ureter	
	10. Sigmoid colon	
	11. Spleen	
	12. Stomach	

Matching

Functions

_____ 13. Concentration of bile

_____ 14. Conjugation of hormones

_____ 15. Exocrine gland

_____ 16. Glycogen production

_____ 17. Major absorption of nutrients

_____ 18. Resorption of electrolytes

_____ 19. Storage and release of blood

Structures

A. Gallbladder
B. Kidney
C. Large intestine
D. Liver
E. Pancreas
F. Small intestine
G. Spleen

Multiple Choice

20. The production of liver bile and pancreatic insulin occurs by what gestational age?
    A. 4 weeks
    B. 12 weeks
    C. 24 weeks
    D. 36 weeks

21. Herniation of the upper stomach through the diaphragm may occur in obese:
    A. adolescents.
    B. Asians.
    C. men.
    D. pregnant women.

22. Which one of the following statements is true concerning liver changes in older adults?
    A. Elongation of the liver occurs
    B. Hepatic blood flow increases
    C. Liver diameter and circumference enlarges
    D. Liver loses some metabolizing ability

HISTORY

23. Cardiac data is collected as part of an abdominal history because heart pain may be:
    A. associated with an incidence of ulcers.
    B. caused by herniation pressure and edema.
    C. perceived as esophagus and stomach pain.
    D. related to congenital abdominal defects.

24. Infant history includes the passage of meconium because an imperforate anus or intestinal obstruction is suspected when a newborn:
    A. fails to pass meconium within 24 hours.
    B. has thick, black tarry stool.
    C. passes light to medium brown stools.
    D. stools more than once in 48 hours.

25. Which of the following is data belonging in a personal and social history?
    A. Abdominal surgery
    B. Familial Mediterranean fever
    C. Recent travel
    D. Urinary incontinence

EXAMINATION

Completion

26. List at least two pieces of equipment needed for the assessment of the abdomen.
    A. _____
    B. _____

27. Describe why you sit to the patient's right to begin abdominal inspection.
    _____

28. Write five ways to make auscultation of the abdomen more accurate and give the rationale for each.

A. _____

_____

B. _____

_____

C. _____

_____

D. _____

_____

E. _____

_____

29. What is accomplished during an abdominal examination by asking the patient to breathe deeply and hold it?

_____

_____

_____

30. Write four ways to make percussion of the abdomen more accurate and give the rationale for each.

A. _____

_____

B. _____

_____

C. _____

_____

D. _____

_____

31. Write four ways to make palpation of the abdomen more accurate and give the rationale for each.

A. _____

_____

B. _____

_____

C. _____

_____

D. _____

_____

FINDINGS

Matching

	Characteristics	Possible Interpretation

_____ 32. Decreased bowel sounds

_____ 33. Generalized symmetric abdominal distention

_____ 34. Glistening abdomen; taut appearance

_____ 35. Umbilical discoloration; Cullen sign

_____ 36. Umbilicus to symphysis abdominal enlargement

_____ 37. Visible peristalsis

A. Ascites
B. Distended bladder
C. Intraabdominal bleeding
D. Obesity
E. Peritonitis
F. Thinness

Multiple Choice

38. Hepatitis B virus is more of a risk for which group of individuals? (p. 481)
    A. Factory workers
    B. Health care professionals
    C. Heterosexual persons
    D. School age children

Situation: You note striae on the abdomen of a 38-year-old nonpregnant women. She is 5'4" tall and weighs 120 pounds. She states that her weight has remained stable over the last few years.

39. What color would you expect her striae to be?
    A. Bluish
    B. Pinkish
    C. Purplish
    D. Whitish

40. Compared to other adults, males and tall individuals usually have a greater:
    A. colon curve.
    B. kidney density.
    C. liver span.
    D. spleen production.

41. What finding is expected from percussing the left lower anterior rib cage and left epigastric region?
    A. Aortic dullness
    B. Gastric bubble
    C. Liver position
    D. Lung resonance

42. Soft, rounded, boggy masses in the cecum or colon areas are most likely:
    A. carcinoma.
    B. feces.
    C. fibroids.
    D. hemorrhoids.

43. Which group has a much higher incidence of gallbladder disease than do other groups?
    A. Alaskan Eskimos
    B. Black Americans
    C. East Indians
    D. Native Americans

44. A finding most indicative of cholecystitis is:
    A. Cullen sign.
    B. Dance sign.
    C. Markle sign.
    D. Murphy sign.

45. The aortic pulse should be:
    A. felt in the anterior direction.
    B. heard but not felt.
    C. in a prominent lateral position.
    D. palpated near the kidney.

46. Sharp pain when McBurney point is palpated is associated with:
    A. appendicitis.
    B. cholecystitis.
    C. intussusception.
    D. kidney stones.

47. Shifting dullness and the puddle sign are maneuvers to assess the presence of:
    A. abdominal fluid.
    B. fetal demise.
    C. hyperactive reflexes.
    D. infected tissue.

48. Which one of the following is correct concerning the mnemonics for "PERITONITIS"?
    A. E = Elevated pulse rate
    B. I = Increasing blood pressure
    C. N = Nausea and vomiting
    D. S = Shifting blood gases

49. Flank tenderness is a finding most associated with:
    A. bowel infarction.
    B. hepatitis.
    C. cholangitis.
    D. renal stones.

50. In the abdomen of a newborn infant, it is common to find:
    A. a concave contour.
    B. dilated superficial veins.
    C. dullness to percussion.
    D. epigastric pulsations.

Situation: A 61-year-old male is admitted with weight loss, fatigue, left lower quadrant abdominal pain, anorexia, and nausea. You find that his bowel sounds are diminished.

51. These findings are most consistent with:
    A. Crohn disease.
    B. diverticulitis.
    C. duodenal ulcers.
    D. ulcerative colitis.

Situation: Examination of a 35-year-old female who presented with fatigue, anorexia, and scleral jaundice determined she had Hepatitis B. She had been exposed to this infection about 100 days previously.

52. Which of the following is a classic finding when examining this patient? (p. 524)
    A. Colicky and severe pain
    B. Enlarged spleen and liver
    C. Generalized rash with itching
    D. Vomiting and indigestion

Situation: Ms. L. describes worsening knifelike pain. She has a history of nausea and vomiting. She reports that she has lost her appetite for sugar and desserts. Her skin appears jaundiced.

53. Which one of the following conditions is consistent with Ms. L.'s history and appearance?
    A. Acute appendicitis
    B. Pancreatitis
    C. Peptic ulcer
    D. Systemic infection

54. Nausea and vomiting are common complaints for a patient who is:
    A. 8 weeks pregnant.
    B. 36 weeks pregnant.
    C. premenopausal.
    D. postmenopausal.

Situation: Ms. O. complains of having about 20 watery, bloody and frequent stools each day. She has lost weight and reports feeling tired.

55. Which of the following conditions is consistent with her signs and symptoms?
    A. Crohn disease
    B. Hiatal hernia
    C. Stomach cancer
    D. Ulcerative colitis

56. Stool that tests guaiac positive is the earliest sign of:
    A. cholecystitis.
    B. colon cancer.
    C. hepatitis.
    D. splenic rupture.

57. A patient with dysuria, nocturia, flank pain, and frequency is most likely suffering from:
    A. glomerulonephritis.
    B. hydronephrosis.
    C. pyelonephritis.
    D. renal failure.

58. Jaundice, hepatomegaly and abdominal distention appearing in an infant 3 weeks of age are consistent with:
    A. biliary atresia.
    B. intussusception.
    C. pyloric stenosis.
    D. necrotizing enterocolitis.

NURSING CONSIDERATIONS

Situation: Ms. B. reports having uncontrolled urine output when she coughs or sneezes. Ms. B. delivered four infants during her childbearing years. After completing her examination, you develop a nursing diagnosis of stress incontinence related to poor muscle tone.

59. Patient teaching may be helpful by encouraging Ms. B. to:
    A. keep her weight slightly above her ideal range.
    B. sit down as much as possible to prevent urinating.
    C. stop aerobic activities that involve stretching.
    D. urinate more frequently to avoid bladder overdistention.

60. Which one of the following defining characteristics is a subjective finding?
    A. Dry skin
    B. Fatigue
    C. Hemoconcentration
    D. Sunken eyeballs

Chapter 14

Female Genitalia

LEARNING OBJECTIVES

After (1) reading the textbook chapter, pages 530–596, (2) studying nursing considerations for Female Genitalia in Part II of this workbook, and (3) completing the following questions, students should be able to:

ANATOMY AND PHYSIOLOGY

1. Recognize anatomy of the female genitalia.
2. Describe physiology of the female genitalia.
3. Identify age and condition variations in the female genitalia.

HISTORY

4. Select patient information relevant to the present problem data of a female genital history.
5. Gather personal and social history data pertinent to a female genital assessment.
6. Collect past medical and family data relevant to a female genital history.
7. Compile age and condition data relevant to a female genital history.

EXAMINATION

8. Identify appropriate equipment for a female genital assessment.

Indicate appropriate techniques for a female genital assessment by:

9. External inspection;
10. Internal inspection;
11. Palpation; and
12. Obtaining smears and cultures.

FINDINGS

13. Recognize expected findings from a female genital examination.
14. Assess variations of minor consequence in female genital findings.
15. Evaluate expected age and condition variations in female genital findings.
16. Assess potential disorders and abnormalities of the female genitalia.
17. Appraise age and condition variations suggesting disorders or abnormalities of the female genitalia.

NURSING CONSIDERATIONS

18. Evaluate cultural factors pertinent to a female genital assessment.
19. Apply critical thinking towards analyzing nursing considerations during a female genital examination.
20. Formulate appropriate nursing diagnoses after completing a female genital assessment.

STUDY FOCUS

Life cycle changes can be readily apparent or not immediately obvious when examining the female genitalia. Particular attention should be given to the age and condition of a woman during this evaluation. Collecting data during a female genitalia assessment requires sensitivity and discretion.

LEARNING ACTIVITIES

ANATOMY AND PHYSIOLOGY

Modified Matching

Structure	***Term***
_____ 1. Bartholin gland opening	"E" = External
_____ 2. Cervical os	"I" = Internal
_____ 3. Endometrium	
_____ 4. Glans of clitoris	
_____ 5. Pouch of Douglas	
_____ 6. Urethral orifice	
_____ 7. Vagina	
_____ 8. Vestibule	

TRUE or Corrected Statement

_____ 9. The <u>urethra</u> is one of the vestibule structures.

_____ 10. The function of <u>Bartholin glands</u> is to drain urethral glands.

_____ 11. The cardinal, uterosacral, round, and broad ligaments of the female pelvis <u>divide the vagina from the bladder</u>.

_____ 12. An ovum travels from the fallopian tubes to the uterus by the <u>force of gravity</u>.

_____ 13. Estrogen and progesterone are hormones secreted by the <u>uterus</u>.

_____ 14. The adnexae of the uterus are composed of the <u>vagina and fundus</u>.

_____ 15. During puberty, vaginal secretions normally become more <u>acidic</u>.

_____ 16. During pregnancy, vaginal secretions <u>turn yellow</u>.

_____ 17. After menopause, <u>adrenal androgens and ovarian testosterone</u> levels decrease.

Completion

18. Use the following terms to label the diagram of the female pelvic organs. Place the correct term in the lettered answer space. Use each term once.

Anterior cul–de–sac
Anus
Bladder
Cervix
Corpus of uterus
External anal sphincter
Fallopian tube
Fundus of uterus
Posterior cul–de–sac
Round ligament
Sacrouterine ligament
Symphysis pubis
Ureter
Urethra
Vagina

A. _____ I. _____
B. _____ J. _____
C. _____ K. _____
D. _____ L. _____
E. _____ M. _____
F. _____ N. _____
G. _____ O. _____
H. _____

HISTORY

19. List five types of data belonging in an obstetric history.

A. _____
B. _____
C. _____
D. _____
E. _____

Situation: Ms. L. has a present problem of vaginal discharge. She states that she takes no medications and does not douche. Her sexual partner has no discharge or symptoms.

20. Describe four types of additional data you would collect related to Ms. L.'s vaginal discharge.

    A. _____
    B. _____
    C. _____
    D. _____

21. State a reason why diabetes is pertinent to the family history about female genitalia.

    _____
    _____
    _____

22. List at least three factors that may be responsible for a child's genital pain.

    A. _____
    B. _____
    C. _____

Matching

Risk Factors

_____ 23. Early menarche; late menopause
_____ 24. Exposure to talc; endometriosis
_____ 25. First coitus at early age; smoking

Cancer

A. Cervical
B. Endometrial
C. Ovarian

EXAMINATION

TRUE or Corrected Statement

_____ 26. When inserting a speculum, move it <u>horizontally</u> until the cervix is seen.

_____ 27. You should rotate the spatula <u>90 degrees</u> when taking a Papanicolaou smear.

_____ 28. <u>A cotton swab</u> is used to collect only endocervical cells.

_____ 29. During <u>bimanual palpation</u>, determine the position of the uterus.

_____ 30. Rectovaginal maneuver is useful for evaluating an <u>anteflexed uterus</u>.

_____ 31. A patient's <u>full bladder</u> may cause her discomfort during an examination.

_____ 32. A speculum should be <u>coated with vaseline</u> before it is inserted and specimens are obtained.

_____ 33. A <u>Gonococcal culture</u> is done before other specimens are collected.

_____ 34. The cervix when grasped should <u>not bend or flex</u>.

_____ 35. A disabled women may be able to assume <u>an "M" or a "V"</u> position for her examination.

FINDINGS

Multiple Choice

36. The perineum of a multiparous woman compared to that of a nulliparous woman is usually:
    A. lighter with wrinkles.
    B. more edematous with skin tags.
    C. smoother and thicker
    D. thinner and more rigid.

Situation: You are examining an adult nonpregnant woman. After inserting the speculum, you observe a normal cervical protrusion.

37. How far into the vagina did this cervix protrude?
    A. 1–3 mm
    B. 4–8 mm
    C. 1–3 cm
    D. 4–7 cm

38. A slit shaped cervical os is most likely related to:
    A. bacterial or fungal infection.
    B. congenital malformation.
    C. mid–cycle cervical change.
    D. trauma from abortion.

39. Adhesions cause:
    A. fixed uterine position.
    B. pinkish cervical color
    C. symmetric vaginal os
    D. vaginal secretions.

40. When examining a woman with a hysterectomy you should:
    A. delete the bimanual and palpation maneuvers.
    B. obtain a Pap smear from the suture line.
    C. omit cultures and specimens from the vagina.
    D. palpate internal areas before inserting the speculum.

41. A prominent labia minora in a newborn:
    A. indicates a maternal infection.
    B. is a normal finding.
    C. suggests ambiguous genitalia.
    D. probably relates to prematurity.

Situation: You are examining a 5-year-old child with a foul vaginal discharge. Her genitals appear normal.

42. What is the most likely cause of her discharge?
    A. Foreign object
    B. Infection
    C. Injury
    D. Ruptured hymen

43. Softness of the cervix is an expected finding for:
    A. adolescent children.
    B. pregnant women.
    C. older adults.
    D. women after menarche.

44. A round pelvis that is typical in 50% of women is:
    A. android.
    B. anthropoid.
    C. gynecoid.
    D. platypelloid.

45. Anthropoid pelvises are more common in:
    A. Asian women.
    B. Black women.
    C. Oriental women.
    D. White women.

46. During pregnancy, myometrial activity results in:
    A. cervical effacement.
    B. Chadwick's sign.
    C. dilation of rugae.
    D. perineal pigmentation.

47. A vagina that becomes narrower, shorter, more constricted and less rugated indicates that a female:
    A. has associated urinary incontinence.
    B. has contracted an STD.
    C. is becoming older.
    D. is lactating after delivery.

48. Before examining an individual with a spinal cord injury, what condition should be assessed and discussed with the patient, if applicable?
    A. Autonomic hyperreflexia
    B. Infected Nabothian cysts
    C. Uterine or rectal prolapse
    D. Vulvar varicosities

Situation: You are examining a woman with edema, weight gain and dysphoria. She describes having occasional food craving.

49. Which condition seems likely?
    A. Candida albicans
    B. Endometriosis
    C. Molluscum contagiosum
    D. Premenstrual syndrome

50. Hemorrhage into the peritoneal cavity is most likely due to:
    A. endometrial hyperplasia.
    B. estrogen therapy.
    C. pelvic inflammatory disease.
    D. ruptured tubal pregnancy.

51. A small midline lower abdominal mass may indicate:
    A. ambiguous genitalia.
    B. atrophic vaginitis.
    C. hydrocolpos.
    D. vulvovaginitis.

Situation: Pelvic examination of the vaginal mucosa of a 28-year-old patient revealed petechiae and paleness. You also observed superficial erosions.

52. These findings are consistent with the diagnosis of:
    A. atrophic vaginitis.
    B. candida infection.
    C. midcycle estradiol fluctuation.
    D. uterine first degree prolapse.

Matching

Descriptions	Terms
_____ 53. Copius, frothy, yellow–green discharge; foul odor	A. *Candida albicans*
_____ 54. Homogeneous grey discharge; foul odor	B. *Chlamydia trachomatis*
_____ 55. Usually asymptomatic	C. *Haemophilus vaginalis*
_____ 56. Usually thick, white, curdy discharge	D. *Neisseria gonorrhoeae*
_____ 57. Yellow-green discharge from cervical os; sometimes absent	E. *Trichomonas vaginalis*

Completion

58. Describe the following conditions in the spaces provided.

A. Condyloma latum: _____

_____

B. Cystocele: _____

_____

C. Ectropion: _____

_____

D. Endometriosis: _____

_____

E. Herpes lesions: _____

_____

F. Myomas: _____

_____

G. PID: _____

_____

H. PMS: _____

_____

I. Ruptured tubal pregnancy: _____

_____

J. Urethral caruncle: _____

_____

K. Uterine prolapse: _____

_____

NURSING CONSIDERATIONS

Situation: You are providing information to Ms. D. about genital self examination. She verbalizes misunderstanding and you determine a nursing diagnosis for Ms. D. of "Knowledge deficit related to unclear understanding of anatomy and physiology."

59. State at least three related factors that should be evaluated to determine the source of Ms. D.'s knowledge deficit.

A. _____
B. _____
C. _____

60. Describe at least three topics that should be addressed during a patient teaching session to promote health and minimize the chance of having recurrent monilial infections.

A. _____
B. _____
C. _____

Chapter 15

Male Genitalia

LEARNING OBJECTIVES

After (1) reading the textbook chapter, pages 597–622, (2) studying nursing considerations for Male Genitalia in Part II of this workbook, and (3) completing the following questions, students should be able to:

ANATOMY AND PHYSIOLOGY

1. Recognize anatomy of the male genitalia.
2. Describe physiology of the male genitalia.
3. Identify age and condition variations in the male genitalia.

HISTORY

4. Select patient information relevant to the present problem data of a male genital history.
5. Gather personal and social history data pertinent to a male genital assessment.
6. Collect past medical and family data relevant to a male genital history.
7. Compile age and condition data relevant to a male genital history.

EXAMINATION

8. Identify appropriate equipment for a male genital assessment.

Indicate appropriate techniques for a male genital assessment by:

9. External inspection;
10. Palpation of external genitalia; and
11. Transillumination of any masses.

FINDINGS

12. Recognize expected findings from a male genital examination.
13. Assess variations of minor consequence in male genital findings.
14. Evaluate expected age and condition variations in male genital findings.
15. Assess potential disorders and abnormalities of the male genitalia.
16. Appraise age and condition variations suggesting disorders or abnormalities of the male genitalia.

NURSING CONSIDERATIONS

17. Evaluate cultural factors pertinent to a male genital assessment.
18. Apply critical thinking towards analyzing nursing considerations during a male genital examination.
19. Formulate appropriate nursing diagnoses after completing a male genital assessment.

STUDY FOCUS

The examination of the male genitalia requires extra care because of the personal nature of this assessment. A quick yet thorough examination is facilitated by correctly learning the anatomy and physiology of the male genitalia. History taking may require a longer time to retrieve information, if the content centers on sensitive issues. Examination techniques follow set protocols. Test your knowledge base by completing the following questions.

LEARNING ACTIVITIES

ANATOMY AND PHYSIOLOGY

Completion

1. Use the following terms to label the diagram of the male pelvic organs. Place the correct term in the lettered answer space. Use each term once.

Anus
Ejaculatory duct
Glans
Prostate gland
Rectum
Seminal vesicle
Symphysis pubis
Testis
Urethra
Urinary bladder

A. _____   F. _____
B. _____   G. _____
C. _____   H. _____
D. _____   I. _____
E. _____   J. _____

114

TRUE or Corrected Statement

_____ 2. The movement of the testes by muscular action regulates <u>ejaculatory flow</u>.

_____ 3. The <u>vas deferens</u> travels through the inguinal canal and unites with the seminal vesicle.

_____ 4. Engorgement of the penis is controlled primarily by <u>the thyroid gland</u>.

_____ 5. Sexual differentiation in the fetus occurs around <u>20 weeks</u> gestation.

_____ 6. The scrotum is more pendulous during <u>the senior years</u>.

HISTORY

_____ 7. The personal history relevant to male genitalia includes mostly data about <u>reproductive function</u>.

_____ 8. Parents of a four year old boy should be asked if he has <u>scrotal swelling</u>.

_____ 9. A risk factor for penile carcinoma is <u>masturbation habits</u>.

_____ 10. A risk factor for testicular carcinoma is <u>cryptorchidism</u>.

EXAMINATION

Matching

Technique

_____ 11. Foreskin retracted
_____ 12. Finger moved along vas deferens
_____ 13. Glands pressed between thumb and forefinger
_____ 14. Mass transilluminated
_____ 15. Testes gently compressed

Purpose

A. Inspecting for urethral discharge
B. Observing for hydrocele
C. Observing for phimosis
D. Palpating for inguinal hernia
E. Palpating for tender testes

FINDINGS

Multiple Choice

16. Balanitis associated with phimosis occurs only in:
    A. adolescent boys.
    B. aging men.
    C. black males.
    D. uncircumcised men.

17. The scrotum is typically:
    A. asymmetric.
    B. bright red.
    C. lightly pigmented.
    D. smoothly textured.

18. Epidermoid cysts on the scrotum occur:
    A. at birth.
    B. in adolescents.
    C. on normal adults.
    D. with sexual diseases.

19. Which of the following testicular characteristics are associated with syphilis or diabetic neuropathy?
    A. Asymmetry and dropping
    B. Bilateral enlargement
    C. Insensitivity to pain
    D. Recession into the abdomen

20. A full term neonate's scrotum is:
    A. fibrotic.
    B. smooth.
    C. pendulous.
    D. without rugae.

21. A flat small scrotum suggests:
    A. cryptorchidism.
    B. hydrocele.
    C. hyperplasia.
    D. varicocele.

22. Young males are more likely to have which type of hernia?
    A. Hiatal
    B. Incarcerated femoral
    C. Indirect inguinal
    D. Umbilical

23. An ovavirus infection resulting in a reddish lesion is:
    A. condyloma acuminatum.
    B. lymphogranuloma venereum.
    C. molluscum contagiosum.
    D. syphilitic chancre.

24. Which lesion is associated with the poxvirus and appears grayish, smooth, and dome shaped?
    A. Condyloma acuminatum
    B. Lymphogranuloma venereum
    C. Molluscum contagiosum
    D. Syphilitic chancre

25. An epididymis with cystic swelling is consistent with:
    A. cystocele.
    B. hydrocele.
    C. spermatocele.
    D. varicocele.

26. An abnormal tortuosity with dilation of the veins within the spermatic cord is a:
    A. cystocele.
    B. hydrocele.
    C. spermatocele.
    D. varicocele.

Situation: A 24-year-old patient has scrotal pain and marked erythema. He may have epididymitis.

27. Which of the following findings would be consistent with epididymitis?
    A. Bacteria in the urine
    B. Pain relief with scrotal elevation
    C. Temperature of 102 degrees Fahrenheit
    D. Uneven scrotal size and shape

28. Hypogonadism and a small scrotum are associated with:
    A. ambiguous genitalia.
    B. hypospadias.
    C. Klinefelter syndrome.
    D. penile carcinoma.

Matching

Characteristics	Interpretations

Characteristics

_____ 29. Associated with mumps

_____ 30. Associated with UTI

_____ 31. Defect in abdominal wall

_____ 32. Deviated penis when erect

_____ 33. Epididymis cystic swelling

_____ 34. Genital warts

_____ 35. Meatus on ventral surface

_____ 36. Painful superficial vesicles

_____ 37. Retracted foreskin

_____ 38. XXY chromosomes

Interpretations

A. Condyloma

B. Epididymitis

C. Hernia

D. Herpes

E. Hypospadias

F. Klinefelter syndrome

G. Orchitis

H. Paraphimosis

I. Spermatocele

J. Peyronie disease

NURSING CONSIDERATIONS

Multiple Choice

Situation: Mr. K. has a positive STS. He states that he doesn't understand how he could have become infected, since he practices safe sex.

39. Your most appropriate initial response to his knowledge deficit is to ask:

A. "Do you know that you have syphilis?"

B. "Do you use intravenous drugs or share needles?"

C. "How many sexual partners have you had recently?"

D. "What methods do you use to practice safe sex?"

40. The effects of illness or medical treatment that changes a person's sexual health is an example of a:

A. chief complaint.

B. defining characteristic.

C. nursing diagnosis.

D. related factor.

LEARNING OBJECTIVES

After (1) reading the textbook chapter, pages 623–643, (2) studying nursing considerations for the Anus, Rectum, and Prostate in Part II of this workbook, and (3) completing the following questions, students should be able to:

ANATOMY AND PHYSIOLOGY

1. Recognize anatomy of the anus, rectum, and prostate.
2. Describe physiology of the anus, rectum, and prostate.
3. Identify age and condition variations in the anus, rectum, and prostate.

HISTORY

4. Select patient information relevant to the present problem data of an anal, rectal, and prostate history.
5. Gather personal and social history data pertinent to an anal, rectal, and prostate assessment.
6. Collect past medical and family data relevant to an anal, rectal, and prostate history.
7. Compile age and condition data relevant to an anal, rectal, and prostate history.

EXAMINATION

8. Identify appropriate equipment for an anal, rectal, and prostate assessment.

Indicate appropriate techniques for an anal, rectal, and prostate assessment by:
9. Inspection of anal and rectal area;
10. Palpation of anal sphincter and perianal area;
11. Palpation of prostate in males; and
12. Inspection of stool.

FINDINGS

13. Recognize expected findings from an anal, rectal, and prostate examination.
14. Assess variations of minor consequence in anal, rectal, and prostate findings.
15. Evaluate expected age and condition variations in anal, rectal and prostate findings.
16. Assess potential disorders and abnormalities of the anus, rectum, and prostate.
17. Appraise age and condition variations suggesting disorders or abnormalities of the anus, rectum, and prostate.

NURSING CONSIDERATIONS

18. Evaluate cultural factors pertinent to an anal, rectal and prostate assessment.
19. Apply critical thinking towards analyzing nursing considerations during an anal, rectal, and prostate examination.
20. Formulate appropriate nursing diagnoses after completing an anal, rectal and prostate assessment.

STUDY FOCUS

Anal and rectal structures are the same for both sexes. Anatomy and physiology of the prostate, of course, is pertinent only to the examination of male patients. As with male and female genitalia, the subject matter of the anal, rectal and prostate history can be embarrassing. Questions must be asked in a manner that will promote an honest, straightforward answer. Test your knowledge of underlying content, examination techniques, and significance of findings by answering the following questions.

LEARNING ACTIVITIES

ANATOMY AND PHYSIOLOGY

Multiple Choice

1. The anal canal is approximately how long?
   A. .05 to 1 cm
   B. 1.5 to 2 cm
   C. 2.5 to 4 cm
   D. 4.5 to 5 cm

2. The lower half of the anal canal is supplied with somatic sensory nerves, making it:
   A. constrict to heat.
   B. dilate during emotional stress.
   C. numb without much feeling.
   D. sensitive to painful stimuli.

3. Which structure is under voluntary control?
   A. Internal smooth muscle
   B. Rectal ampulla
   C. Striated external sphincter
   D. Upper anal canal

4. Which structure has mostly somatic sensory nerves?
   A. Lower half of canal
   B. Prostate gland
   C. Sigmoid colon
   D. Superior rectal valve

5. The rectum is approximately how long?
   A. 8 cm
   B. 10 cm
   C. 12 cm
   D. 14 cm

6. The median lobe of the prostate is composed of glandular tissue and contains:
   A. collecting ducts.
   B. myelinated tubules.
   C. secretory alveoli.
   D. terminal lobes.

7. Collagen replaces the muscular component of the prostate during:
   A. adolescence.
   B. childhood.
   C. infancy.
   D. older adulthood.

8. The sudden appearance and later spontaneous disappearance of hemorrhoids is typically found in:
   A. Native Indians.
   B. newborn infants.
   C. pregnant women.
   D. older men.

HISTORY

Completion

9. What three conditions in family members are relevant to a family history?
   A. _____
   B. _____
   C. _____

   Situation: Mr. N. states that he thinks he has a hemorrhoid, because he noticed some rectal bleeding.

10. Describe at least four types of information you would gather during his history.
    A. _____
    B. _____
    C. _____
    D. _____

11. List three congenital conditions of the anus, rectum, and prostate relevant to the history of an infant.
    A. _____
    B. _____
    C. _____

EXAMINATION

12. List three types of equipment used during an anal, rectal, and prostate examination.

A. _____

B. _____

C. _____

13. Explain how to examine the anal canal correctly. Include description of patient position, equipment, and technique to be used.

_____

_____

_____

_____

14. Describe how you would examine the anal ring, rectal wall, and prostate. State how you would palpate for a perianal abscess.

_____

_____

_____

_____

15. List at least two characteristics that should be described after you palpate the prostate gland through the anterior rectal wall.

A. _____

B. _____

Matching

Technique	*Examination Rationale*
_____ 16. Bidigital palpation of perianal tissue	A. Appraising newborn patency
_____ 17. Lubricated catheter 1cm into rectum	B. Assessing cervix or prostate
_____ 18. Palpation of anterior rectal wall	C. Detecting perianal abscess
_____ 19. Patient bears down on examiner's finger	D. Estimating sphincter tone
_____ 20. Rotation of forefinger inside anus	E. Evaluating anal ring

FINDINGS

TRUE or Corrected Statement

_____ 21. Fissures, abscesses and pilonidal cysts cause <u>bulging and wrinkling</u>.

_____ 22. An <u>inverted cervix</u> is a sign of a chronic debilitating disease.

_____ 23. <u>Viscous, occult positive</u> stool is a normal newborn finding.

_____ 24. A smooth, large, rubbery prostate is a common finding in <u>adolescents</u>.

_____ 25. <u>Chronic prostatitis</u> is usually asymptomatic.

_____ 26. <u>Blue, shiny masses</u> around the anus are common findings late in pregnancy.

_____ 27. Incomplete bladder emptying, frequency, and dysuria are findings consistent with <u>prostatic carcinoma</u>.

Matching

	Description	Condition
_____	28. Anorectal fetal malformation	A. Anorectal fissure
_____	29. Boggy, enlarged prostate	B. BPH
_____	30. Chronic perianal skin inflammation	C. Chronic prostatitis
_____	31. Dimple with sinus tract opening	D. Hemorrhoids
_____	32. Erythema of the anus	E. Imperforate anus
_____	33. Rosette–looking mucosa	F. Perianal abscess
_____	34. Sessile polypoid mass	G. Pilonidal cyst
_____	35. Tear in anal mucosa	H. Pruritus ani
_____	36. Urinary hesitancy and dribbling	I. Rectal cancer
_____	37. Varicose veins	J. Rectal prolapse

NURSING CONSIDERATIONS

Completion

38. List at least two subjective and two objective defining characteristics for constipation.
SUBJECTIVE
   A. _____
   B. _____
OBJECTIVE
   C. _____
   D. _____

39. State at least three potential related factors to a nursing diagnosis of "Bowel Incontinence."
   A. _____
   B. _____
   C. _____

Situation: You have completed a history on Mr. J. and note that his diet is high in fat and low in fiber. He reports drinking few fluids, except for beer and milk. He states that he has bowel movements about twice a week.

40. Compose a nursing diagnosis pertinent to Mr. J.'s condition.

_____

_____

Chapter 17

Musculoskeletal System

LEARNING OBJECTIVES

After (1) reading the textbook chapter, pages 644–711, (2) studying nursing considerations for the Musculoskeletal System in Part II of this workbook, and (3) completing the following questions, students should be able to:

ANATOMY AND PHYSIOLOGY

1. Recognize anatomy of the musculoskeletal system.
2. Describe physiology of the musculoskeletal system.
3. Identify age and condition variations in the musculoskeletal system.

HISTORY

4. Select patient information relevant to the present problem data of a musculoskeletal history.
5. Gather personal and social history data pertinent to a musculoskeletal assessment.
6. Collect past medical and family data relevant to a musculoskeletal history.
7. Compile age and condition data relevant to a musculoskeletal history.

EXAMINATION

8. Identify appropriate equipment for a musculoskeletal assessment.

Indicate appropriate techniques for a musculoskeletal assessment by:

9. Inspection;
10. Palpation;
11. Testing; and
12. Measurement.

FINDINGS

13. Recognize expected findings from a musculoskeletal examination.
14. Assess variations of minor consequence in musculoskeletal findings.
15. Evaluate expected age and condition variations in musculoskeletal findings.
16. Assess potential disorders and abnormalities of the musculoskeletal system.
17. Appraise age and condition variations suggesting disorders or abnormalities of the musculoskeletal system.

NURSING CONSIDERATIONS

18. Evaluate cultural factors pertinent to a musculoskeletal assessment.
19. Apply critical thinking towards analyzing nursing considerations during a musculoskeletal examination.
20. Formulate appropriate nursing diagnoses after completing a musculoskeletal assessment.

STUDY FOCUS

Mobility and stability are achieved by the musculoskeletal system. A thorough history and examination distinguishes normal findings from those indicating abnormalities. Metabolic disorders, injuries, and other defects or diseases may result in disability and require additional assessment. Remember to assess the bony structure in unison with its associated muscles, tendons, ligaments and cartilage. Hematologic and neurologic data is also important to a musculoskeletal examination. Apply your knowledge by completing the following exercises.

LEARNING ACTIVITIES

ANATOMY AND PHYSIOLOGY

Matching

Movement

_____ 1. Flexion and extension in one plane
_____ 2. Gliding only
_____ 3. Rotation only
_____ 4. Two planes at right angles with no axial rotation
_____ 5. Two planes at right angles with no radial rotation
_____ 6. Wide range in all planes

Joint Types

A. Ball and Socket
B. Condyloid
C. Gliding
D. Hinge
E. Pivot
F. Saddle

Location

_____ 7. Atlantoaxis
_____ 8. Carpal–metacarpal thumb joint
_____ 9. Elbow
_____ 10. Hip
_____ 11. Intervertebral
_____ 12. Wrist between radius and carpals

Joint Types

A. Ball and Socket
B. Condyloid
C. Gliding
D. Hinge
E. Pivot
F. Saddle

13. What is the difference in process between bone growth in the long bones and the small short bones?

_____

_____

_____

_____

14. What is the effect of softened cartilage and elasticized ligaments on the joints of pregnant women, and which joints are affected during pregnancy?

_____

_____

_____

5. What happens to muscle mass, tone, and strength as people age?

_____

_____

_____

Completion

16. Use the following terms to label the diagram of the muscles. Place the correct term in the lettered answer space. Use each term once.

Clavicle
Deltoid
External oblique
Internal oblique
Pectoralis major
Rectus abdominis
Sternocleidomastoid
Transversus abdominis
Trapezius

A. _____   F. _____

B. _____   G. _____

C. _____   H. _____

D. _____   I. _____

E. _____

Multiple Choice

17. The functions of the musculoskeletal system include vital organ protection, mineral storage, and:
    A. blood cell production.
    B. breakdown of toxins.
    C. lymphatic drainage.
    D. progesterone secretion.

18. Which group of vertebrae are the most mobile?
    A. Cervical
    B. Lumbar
    C. Sacral
    D. Thoracic

19. What structure within the knee provides for anterior and posterior stability?
    A. Articulated patella
    B. Cruciate ligaments
    C. Medial epicondyle
    D. Vastus medialis

20. The number of muscle fibers ultimately develops:
    A. at birth.
    B. by age 20.
    C. during puberty.
    D. in utero.

21. Ligaments are stronger than bone until:
    A. birth.
    B. older adulthood.
    C. pregnancy.
    D. puberty.

HISTORY

Completion

Situation: Ms. R., age 55, has a chief complaint of stiff knees in the morning.
Name three examples of information you should obtain from Ms. R. related to each of the following categories.

22. Character
    A. _____
    B. _____
    C. _____

23. Associated events
    A. _____
    B. _____
    C. _____

24. Temporal factors
    A. _____
    B. _____
    C. _____

25. Efforts to treat
    A. _____
    B. _____
    C. _____

26. Write one reason for asking the following questions during Ms. R's past medical history.
    A. Have you ever had neurologic disorders?

    _____
    _____

    B. Were you born with any bone defects?

    _____
    _____

27. Explain why it is useful to know whether Ms. R.'s mother had foot deformities.

    _____
    _____

28. Describe at least two types of information important to seek about the joints of all people in
    Ms. R.'s age group.
    A. _____

    _____
    B. _____

    _____

Situation: Mr. M., age 68, has no complaints of musculoskeletal disorder. You are reviewing his musculoskeletal system during a preventive medical check-up.

29. Opposite each data category give at least one reason why this information is needed for Mr. M's musculoskeletal system.

Data	*Reason*
A. Past employment	A. _____
	_____
B. Exercise	B. _____
	_____
C. Elimination	C. _____
	_____
D. Aspirin	D. _____
	_____
E. Communication	E. _____
	_____
F. Diet	F. _____
	_____

EXAMINATION

Multiple Choice

30. Which technique is most useful for assessing joint symmetry?
    A. Inspection
    B. Palpation
    C. Percussion
    D. Use of joint calipers

31. A goniometer is used to assess:
    A. bone maturity.
    B. joint proportions.
    C. joint range of motion.
    D. muscle contractions.

32. The extension of the patient's head against the examiner's hand is a test of:
    A. cervical spine alignment.
    B. passive range of motion.
    C. temporalis muscle strength.
    D. trapezius muscle strength.

33. What examination technique is used to assess the sternoclavicular joint, acromioclavicular joint, clavicle, scapulae, coracoid process, greater trochanter of the humerus and the biceps groove?
    A. Auscultation
    B. Inspection
    C. Palpation
    D. Percussion

34. A technique used to detect a torn meniscus is the:
    A. Drawer test.
    B. McMurray test.
    C. Thomas test.
    D. Trendelenburg test.

35. Which procedure to detect hip dislocation is performed at each infant examination during the first year of life?
    A. Ballottement maneuvers
    B. Barlow Ortolani maneuver
    C. Range of flexion
    D. Thomas McMurray assessment

FINDINGS

Completion

36. List five findings that you should note about a patient's musculoskeletal system.
    A. _____
    B. _____
    C. _____
    D. _____
    E. _____

37. List three types of data you would collect about a patient with temporomandibular joint clicks.
    A. _____
    B. _____
    C. _____

38. What are two findings that suggest a disorder of the popliteal space?
    A. _____
    B. _____

39. What are two expected findings from palpation of the tibiofemoral joint?

    A. _____

    B. _____

40. What three palpation findings suggest tibiofemoral joint problems?

    A. _____

    B. _____

    C. _____

41. When examining a newborn's knees, what characteristic would you expect?

    _____

42. Why do pregnant women have lordosis and cervical flexion?

    _____

Multiple Choice

43. Which group of women rarely develops serious osteoporosis due to bones that are more dense?

    A. American Indians

    B. Blacks

    C. East Indians

    D. Whites

44. A risk factor that may facilitate a sports injury is:

    A. overuse of fluids.

    B. preconditioning exercises.

    C. rapid adolescent growth.

    D. wearing protective clothing.

45. A more prominent gluteal muscle may promote lordosis in:

    A. Asian women.

    B. black women.

    C. newborn infants.

    D. thin men.

46. Tinel sign is associated with:

    A. carpal tunnel syndrome.

    B. osteitis deformans.

    C. radial head subluxation.

    D. talipes equinovarus.

47. Physical examination of an elderly woman with advanced osteoporosis commonly reveals a/an:
    A. decrease in weight.
    B. expansion of bone density.
    C. increase in height.
    D. spinal deformity.

48. Which group of infants often has advanced motor development over Caucasian Americans under the age of three years?
    A. Asian Americans
    B. Black Americans
    C. Danish Americans
    D. German Americans

49. Which group is susceptible to the preventable condition of subluxation of the head of the radius?
    A. Adolescents
    B. Older adults
    C. Pregnant women
    D. Toddlers

50. An increase in the lumbosacral curve is a common finding for:
    A. adolescent boys.
    B. newborn infants.
    C. older adults.
    D. pregnant women.

Matching

Characteristic	*Possible Interpretation*
_____ 51. Bone mass decrease	A. Ankylosing spondylitis
_____ 52. Deposits of urate salts	B. Carpal tunnel syndrome
_____ 53. Excessive bone formation	C. Gout
_____ 54. Eventual spinal deformity	D. Paget disease
_____ 55. Lateral spin curvature	E. Scoliosis
_____ 56. Nocturnal hand tingling	F. Spina bifida
_____ 57. Neural tube defect	G. TMJ
_____ 58. Unilateral facial pain	H. Osteoporosis

Description	Associated Term
_____ 59. Anterior serratus is denervated	A. Kyphosis
_____ 60. Boutonniere and spindle shaped deformities	B. Nulliparity
_____ 61. Collapsed vertebra and gibbus	C. Obesity
_____ 62. Risk factor for osteoarthritis	D. Rheumatoid arthritis
_____ 63. Risk factor for osteoporosis	E. Winged scapula

Condition	Disorder
_____ 64. Absence of clavicles	A. Cleidocranial dysostosis
_____ 65. Bilateral palmar fascia defect	B. Dupuytren contracture
_____ 66. Degeneration of muscle fibers	C. Muscular dystrophy
_____ 67. Injured joint ligament	D. Osteomyelitis
_____ 68. Infection of a bone	E. Sprain

NURSING CONSIDERATIONS

Multiple Choice

69. Which nursing diagnosis is most appropriate to the definition of: "The state in which an individual experiences a limitation of ability for independent physical movement"?
    A. Activity disability from limitations
    B. Impaired physical mobility
    C. Instability related to spasms
    D. Limited range of motion

70. Related factors of inflammation, muscle spasm, pressure and trauma are most likely associated with a nursing diagnosis of:
    A. anxiety.
    B. impaired skin integrity.
    C. knowledge deficit.
    D. pain.

Chapter 18

Neurologic System and Mental Status

LEARNING OBJECTIVES

After (1) reading the textbook chapter, pages 712–774, (2) studying nursing considerations for the Neurologic System in part II of this workbook, and (3) completing the following questions, students should be able to:

ANATOMY AND PHYSIOLOGY

1. Recognize anatomy of the neurologic system.
2. Describe physiology of the neurologic system.
3. Identify age and condition variations in the neurologic system.

HISTORY

4. Select patient information relevant to the present problem data of a neurologic history.
5. Gather personal and social history data pertinent to a neurologic assessment.
6. Collect past medical and family data relevant to a neurologic history.
7. Compile age and condition data relevant to a neurologic history.

EXAMINATION

8. Identify appropriate equipment for a neurologic assessment.

Indicate appropriate techniques for a neurologic assessment by:

9. Inspection and testing mental and behavior abilities;
10. Cranial nerve and sensory testing;
11. Proprioception and cerebellar function testing; and
12. Reflex testing.

FINDINGS

13. Recognize expected findings from a neurologic examination.
14. Assess variations of minor consequence in neurologic findings.
15. Evaluate expected age and condition variations in neurologic findings.
16. Assess potential disorders and abnormalities of the neurologic system.
17. Appraise age and condition variations suggesting disorders or abnormalities of the neurologic system.

NURSING CONSIDERATIONS

18. Evaluate cultural factors pertinent to a neurologic assessment.
19. Apply critical thinking towards analyzing nursing considerations during a neurologic examination.
20. Formulate appropriate nursing diagnoses after completing a neurologic assessment.

STUDY FOCUS

An intact neurologic system allows the body to function and perform tasks. Voluntary and involuntary activities must be assessed with their corresponding motor, sensory, cognitive, psychologic and behavioral elements. Review the anatomy and physiology of the brain and spinal cord. Remember to evaluate developmental changes as part of a neurologic examination. There is a unique relationship between motor functioning and mental capabilities. While reviewing the usual findings from a nervous system examination, also consider potential pathology that can alter consciousness, muscle tone, behavior and other mental and neurologic abilities.

LEARNING ACTIVITIES

ANATOMY AND PHYSIOLOGY

Completion

1. Opposite each structure write at least one associated function in the blanks to the right.

Structure	Function
A. Glossopharyngeal (IX)	A. _____
B. Cerebellum	B. _____
C. Acoustic (VIII)	C. _____
D. Pyramidal tract	D. _____
E. Temporal lobe	E. _____
F. Parietal lobe	F. _____
G. Abducens (VI)	G. _____
H. Spinothalamic tract	H. _____
I. Trigeminal (V)	I. _____
J. Occipital lobe	J. _____
K. Facial (VII)	K. _____
L. Anterior horn	L. _____

2. Use the following terms to label this diagram of the diencephalon structures and location of cranial nerve roots.

Abducens (VI)
Accessory (XI)
Acoustic (VIII)
Cerebellum
Cerebral peduncle
Cerebrum
Facial (VII)
Glossopharyngeal (IX)
Hypoglossal (XII)
Hypothalamus
Oculomotor (III)
Olfactory (I)
Optic (II)
Pituitary gland
Thalamus
Trigeminal (V)
Trochlear (IV)
Vagus (X)

A. _____   J. _____
B. _____   K. _____
C. _____   L. _____
D. _____   M. _____
E. _____   N. _____
F. _____   O. _____
G. _____   P. _____
H. _____   Q. _____
I. _____   R. _____

Multiple Choice

3. Which area of the brain is responsible for interpreting tactile sensations?
    A. Frontal lobe
    B. Occipital lobe
    C. Parietal lobe
    D. Temporal lobe

4. The state of consciousness is controlled in the brainstem area of the:
   A. corpus callosum.
   B. hypothalamus.
   C. pituitary gland.
   D. thalamus.

5. Which structure is responsible for sexual development and behavior?
   A. Epithalamus
   B. Pituitary gland
   C. Pons
   D. Thalamus

6. Motor maturation proceeds from:
   A. centrally to peripherally.
   B. head to toe.
   C. laterally to medially.
   D. pedal to cephalic.

7. Why do the elderly tend to have deliriums when they become acutely ill?
   A. Hypothalamic-pituitary hormones change with age.
   B. Intelligence decreases with age.
   C. Neurotransmitter metabolism declines with age.
   D. Serotonin production is facilitated by illness.

HISTORY

Completion

8. Name four neurologic disorders that are known to be hereditary.
   A. _____
   B. _____
   C. _____
   D. _____

9. Opposite each problem write at least two items of additional data that you would collect, besides the date of onset.

Problem	Additional Data Needed
A. Falling during walking	A.1. _____
	2. _____
B. Dizziness	B.1. _____
	2. _____
C. Swallowing difficulty	C.1. _____
	2. _____
D. Numbness	D.1. _____
	2. _____

10. Explain the relevance of deformitites and congenital anomalies to the neurologic past medical history.

_____

_____

11. Opposite each condition write at least one reason, other than heredity, for including each of the following in a family history.

Condition	*Reason for Inclusion*
A. Headaches; gait disorders	A. _____
	_____
B. Mental illness	B. _____
	_____
C. Learning disorders	C. _____
	_____

12. Name at least five types of information needed for the neurologic history of infants.

A. _____

B. _____

C. _____

D. _____

E. _____

EXAMINATION

TRUE or Corrected Statement

_____ 13. <u>Sensory function</u> is assessed when you test a patient's ability to perceive touch, vibration and position changes.

_____ 14. You are testing <u>vagus nerve function</u>, when you ask a patient the meaning of a fable or proverb.

_____ 15. The finger to nose test evaluates <u>deep tendon reflexes.</u>

_____ 16. Balance is initially assessed with the <u>Romberg test</u>.

_____ 17. The <u>Kernig and Brudzinski</u> test is used to qualify consciousness.

_____ 18. You can evaluate one function of the <u>cerebellum</u> by observing whether or not a newborn has coordinated sucking and swallowing.

FINDINGS

Matching

	Characteristic	*Infant Reflex*
_____	19. Downward curled toes	A. Galant
_____	20. Fencing posture	B. Moro
_____	21. Flexion of hips and knees	C. Placing
_____	22. Initial symmetric abduction	D. Plantar grasp
_____	23. Trunk incurvature	E. Tonic neck

	Infant Behaviors	*Ages*
_____	24. Babbling, cooing	A. Birth
_____	25. Glabella reflex	B. 2 to 3 months
_____	26. Hand to hand transfers	C. 3 to 4 months
_____	27. Mama, Dada	D. 4 to 6 months
_____	28. Parachute reflex	E. 6 to 8 months
_____	29. Social smiling	F. 9 to 10 months

Completion

30. Name four findings that indicate a healthy sensorium.

    A. _____

    B. _____

    C. _____

    D. _____

31. State the most important expected finding from a test of reflexes in any extremity.

    _____

32. Name two instances in which Babinski sign is a normal finding.

    A. _____

    B. _____

33. Describe what a patient should feel when you strike a tuning fork and place it directly on a bony prominence.

    _____

34. Name six functional behaviors that you would expect in a healthy newborn.

    A. _____

    B. _____

    C. _____

    D. _____

    E. _____

    F. _____

Multiple Choice

35. Confusion with disordered perceptions and decreased attention span is a sign of:

    A. confusion.

    B. delirium.

    C. lethargy.

    D. stupor.

Situation: Ms. S. is nonresponsive. Her breathing is regular. When you call her name, she moves. Ms. S. groans when she experiences painful stimuli.

36. Ms. S.'s level of consciousness is:
    A. confused.
    B. delirious.
    C. lethargic.
    D. stuporous.

37. A patient who has difficulty writing or drawing is more likely to have which condition?
    A. Cerebral disfunction
    B. Organic brain syndrome
    C. Peripheral neuropathy
    D. Psychiatric hallucinations

Situation: A patient has neurologic damage to the brain regions that control speech and language. This patient cannot verbally communicate.

38. What term would you expect to see documented?
    A. Aphasic
    B. Amusic
    C. Dysarthric
    D. Dysphonic

39. What cranial nerve would you further evaluate, if a patient cannot shrug his or her shoulders against resistance?
    A. CN I, olfactory
    B. CN V, trigeminal
    C. CN IX, glossopharyngeal
    D. CN XI, spinal accessory

40. A patient has impaired pain sensation, so you decide to perform additional tests with:
    A. hot and cold water.
    B. radiopaque dye.
    C. transilluminating light.
    D. ultrasonic waves.

41. Which cranial nerve requires further evaluation when a patient cannot discern between sour and bitter flavors?
    A. CN I, olfactory
    B. CN V, trigeminal
    C. CN IX, glossopharyngeal
    D. CN XI, spinal accessory

Situation: Mr. M. has difficulty with his heel to toe walking ability. He states that he has recently had problems maintaining his balance.

42. It is most important to evaluate Mr. M.'s:

    A. deep tendon reflexes.

    B. mental and emotional status.

    C. proprioception and cerebellar function.

    D. tactile, touch and taste tests.

43. A normal finding from squeezing a biceps muscle is:

    A. burning.

    B. discomfort.

    C. tingling.

    D. warmth.

Matching

Characteristics	*Gait*
_____ 44. Affected leg is stiff	A. Ataxia
_____ 45. Heel stamps on ground	B. Dystonic
_____ 46. Jerky dancing movements	C. Dystrophic
_____ 47. Lordosis is often present	D. Spastic diplegia
_____ 48. Unable to walk on heel	E. Spastic hemiparesis
_____ 49. Uncontrolled falling occurs	F. Steppage
_____ 50. Walks with short steps	G. Tabetic

Finding	*Neurologic Disorder*
_____ 51. Coarse tremors of tongue	A. Delirium tremens
_____ 52. Episodes of clonic contractions	B. Huntington chorea
_____ 53. Fever, loss of consciousness	C. Meningitis
_____ 54. Loss of discriminatory sensation	D. Multiple sclerosis
_____ 55. Rapid, short, shuffling steps	E. Parkinson disease
_____ 56. Spastic leg weakness, ataxia	F. Peripheral neuropathy
_____ 57. Twitching, mental deterioration	G. Seizures

NURSING CONSIDERATIONS

Completion

Situation: Mr. H., age 45, has been working two jobs and verbalizes that he remains tired. He is concerned about his decreased ability to think and remember things. Mr. H. reports being more short tempered than ever before.

58. Compose an appropriate nursing diagnosis.

_____

_____

59. State at least one defining characteristic that could be an expected subjective finding for someone with impaired verbal communication related to ineffective listening skills?

_____

_____

60. List at least two kinesthetic related factors pertinent to a nursing diagnosis of "Sensory-Perceptual alterations: Kinesthetic, tactile."

A. _____

B. _____

Chapter 19

Putting It All Together

LEARNING OBJECTIVES

After (1) reading the textbook chapter, pages 775–806, (2) reviewing the nursing process presented in Part II of this workbook, and (3) completing the following questions, students should be able to:

ASSESSMENT GUIDELINES

1. Delineate guidelines to be followed while conducting a history and physical examination.
2. Evaluate patient and health provider reliability during the collection of subjective and objective data.
3. Analyze the use of machines, equipment, and supplies during a physical examination.

EXAMINATION STEPS

4. Indicate correct inspection, palpation, percussion, auscultation, and measuring techniques for examining patient systems.
5. Identify appropriate steps for examining systems when patients are in a sitting, supine, standing, and lithotomy, knee–chest or similar positions.
6. Appraise techniques for seeing, hearing, musculoskeletal, and neurologic testing.
7. Select modifications for examining patients throughout the life cycle.
8. Describe adjustments that can be made when examining persons with disabilities.

EVALUATION

9. Appraise factors that influence patients' perceptions of their symptoms.
10. Assess methods for evaluating the examination skills of students.
11. Analyze factors involved in postexamination decision making.

STUDY FOCUS

Subjective information collected during the history and objective data gained from performing a physical examination are combined to provide a more complete picture of a patient's health. History and physical findings must be analyzed together. While completing the following questions, focus on content that will most help you gather and report your findings from a patient assessment. Remember to be flexible, yet thorough and organized.

LEARNING ACTIVITIES
ASSESSMENT GUIDELINES

Multiple Choice

1. An illness when understood in human terms and expressed by the patient should be described within which category of the history?
   A. Laboratory and test section
   B. Past disease data
   C. Subjective findings
   D. Systemic assessment

2. Patient dissatisfaction is best minimized if the health care provider:
   A. assumes a hurried manner.
   B. conveys feelings of disgust.
   C. encourages patient questions.
   D. keeps the patient waiting.

   Situation: A 50-year-old man is being seen for his employment physical. He states that he is healthy and hates being "poked and picked at."
3. Your best response would be to:
   A. explain that his feelings are normal.
   B. immediately back away from him.
   C. make a joke about his insecurity.
   D. perform a quicker that usual examination.

4. Which one of the following patient characteristics is most likely to limit the collection of reliable data?
   A. Alert and oriented to date and place
   B. Appropriate mental status and neural responses
   C. Culturally different from health care provider
   D. Sensory assessment results within normal range

Completion

5. Describe the relationship between taking the history and performing the physical examination.

   _____
   _____
   _____
   _____

6. List at least two things you should explain to patients.

A. _____

B. _____

_____

7. Explain at least two aspects of the examiner's behavior that facilitates patient assessment.

A. _____

B. _____

8. Explain at least two guideines concerning the patient during an examination.

A. _____

B. _____

9. Describe at least two human skills that are needed for optimally assessing patient status.

A. _____

B. _____

10. Identify at least two technologic methods that provide details unavailable from examination alone.

A. _____

B. _____

EXAMINATION STEPS

Modified Matching

Place "Front", "Behind", or "F & B" on each blank line to indicate hte examiner position when assessing the seated patient.

Front = Examiner in front of seated patient

Behind = Examiner in back of seated patient

F & B = Examiner stands both in front and in back of patient

_____ 11. Palpate lacrimal apparatus

_____ 12. Palpate auricle

_____ 13. Palpate and percuss costovertebral angle

_____ 14. Palpate superficial cervical chain

_____ 15. Percuss for diaphragmatic excursion

_____ 16. Percuss systematically for resonance

_____ 17. Palpate for tactile fremitus

_____ 18. Assess olfactory function

_____ 19. Inspect configuration of skull

_____ 20. Palpate scapular and subscapular nodes

_____ 21. Note anteroposterior pillars

_____ 22. Palpate temporomandibular joint

_____ 23. Palpate epitrochlear nodes

_____ 24. Auscultate systematically for breath sounds

Matching

	Examination Technique		Potential Finding

_____ 25. Auscultate renal and femoral arteries for:

_____ 26. Auscultate all abdominal quadrants for:

_____ 27. Palpate midline for:

_____ 28. Palpate right costal margin for:

_____ 29. Percuss all abdominal quadrants for:

_____ 30. Percuss left midaxillary line for:

Potential Finding
A. aortic pulsation.
B. bowel sounds.
C. bruits.
D. liver border.
E. splenic dullness.
F. tone.

Neurologic Test

_____ 31. Deep tendon reflexes

_____ 32. Sensory function

_____ 33. Two–point discrimination

_____ 34. Vibratory sensation

Anatomic Site
A. ankles, wrists
B. biceps, patellar
C. forehead, paranasal sinus
D. palms, thighs

Multiple Choice

35. An assessment of the retinal surface is part of a/an:
    A. corneal reflex test.
    B. ophthalmoscopic examination.
    C. otoscopic inspection.
    D. Rosenbaum screening.

36. Inspection of jugular venous pulsations and measurement of jugular venous pressure is done with the patient in which position?
    A. Completey supine
    B. Lithotomy or knee chest
    C. Reclined 45 degrees
    D. Standing upright

37. By 40 weeks of gestation, newborns should have:
    A. breast nodules less than 3 mm.
    B. lanugo covering back and legs.
    C. one transverse sole crease.
    D. scrotum covered with rugae.

38. Tactile fremitus and cranial nerves IX, X, and XII are best evaluated when the infant is:
    A. burping.
    B. crying.
    C. sleeping.
    D. sucking.

39. Each side of an infant's mouth should be stroked to evaluate:
   A. nystagmus.
   B. patency of choanae.
   C. rooting reflex.
   D. tonic neck.

40. Evaluating an infant's placing reflex is part of the:
   A. Dobowitz assessment.
   B. lower extremities examination.
   C. neurologic assessment.
   D. upper extremities examination.

41. A child's muscle strength may be evaluated when the child:
   A. "blows out" the otoscope.
   B. clings to mother with fear.
   C. plays on the floor.
   D. stands on the scale.

42. Palpation of the dorsalis pedis pulse is done when the child is:
   A. bending over examination table.
   B. on the parent's lap.
   C. standing on one foot.
   D. supine with loosened diaper.

Situation: A three year old boy is crying and says that he doesn't want a shot. His mother is holding him and explains that you are just going to look at him.
43. One of the best ways to decrease anxiety in this child before his examination is to:
   A. apply a mummy restraint.
   B. hide the equipment from him.
   C. hold his head down.
   D. let him play with the flashlight.

44. Which one of the following items is most relevant to the evaluation of an older adult?
   A. Developmental scoring
   B. Functional assessment
   C. Gestational history
   D. Physical measurements

45. When examining a disabled person, it is most appropriate to:
   A. adjust your examination sequence as needed.
   B. maintain a rigid examination protocol.
   C. omit aspects of the history and examination.
   D. refuse to perform an examination without help.

EVALUATION

TRUE or Corrected Statement

_____ 46. Illness without disease is usually related to <u>subjective</u> perceptions.

_____ 47. One method for evaluating student examiners is to assess whether or not students <u>repeat patient statements</u>.

_____ 48. Postexamination decision making may include the use of algorithms and <u>hypotheses</u>.

_____ 49. When a patient has not been compliant with instructions, an examiner should <u>reprimand the patient</u>.

_____ 50. Illness is almost always related to a <u>single</u> phenomenon.

LEARNING OBJECTIVES

After (1) reading the textbook chapter, pages 807–827, and (2) completing the following questions, students should be able to:

SURVEYS

1. Identify the components of the primary survey.
2. Indicate the components of the secondary survey.
3. Describe appropriate re–evaluation measures for emergency patients.
4. Delineate the use and meaning of the mnemonics: ABCs, AVPU, and AMPLE.

INTERPRETATION AND DOCUMENTATION

5. Differentiate symptoms associated with injuries and trauma.
6. Recognize signs and symptoms of life–threatening conditions.
7. Appraise findings that indicate the need for emergency intervention for infants and children.
8. Describe documentation procedures for emergency patients.

STUDY FOCUS

The history and physical examination process is conducted with patients who have chronic conditions. It is also done to assess health risks and prevent illness. There is yet another situation when physical examination skills are required. The following questions center on assessment skills needed for patient's with acute disorders and emergency conditions.

LEARNING ACTIVITIES

SURVEYS

Completion

1. Describe what each of the following letters represents for assessing and managing an emergency patient.

A: _____

B: _____

C: _____

D: _____

E: _____

2. During the secondary survey, a history should be done that includes "AMPLE" information. Describe what each of these letters represents.

A: _____

M: _____

P: _____

L: _____

E: _____

3. State what each "AVPU" letter represents, and describe how this mnemonic is used to assess a patient's level of responsiveness.

A: _____

V: _____

P: _____

U: _____

Multiple Choice

4. The primary survey, or assessment of the ABC's, should take approximately how long in a stable patient?
   A. 30 seconds
   B. 60 seconds
   C. 2 minutes
   D. 5 minutes

5. The primary survey should be performed every:
   A. 30 seconds
   B. 60 seconds
   C. 2 minutes
   D. 5 minutes

Situation: Mr. M., a trauma patient, verbalizes severe rib pain. His vital signs are within normal range. His coworker states that Mr. M. was accidently hit in his torso with a large pipe.

6. The presence of which finding is most important to monitor throughout Mr. M.'s secondary survey?
    A. Clubbed fingers
    B. Flail chest
    C. Pupil constriction
    D. Rebound tenderness

Situation: You are conducting a secondary survey of Ms. L. and find that she has a systolic blood pressure below 80 mm. Her color is pale, although her respiratory rate is within normal range.

7. Which one of the following conditions was a likely finding during Ms. L.'s primary survey?
    A. Bilaterally equal radial pulses
    B. Pulse rate within normal range
    C. Radial pulse cannot be palpated
    D. Strong, bounding radial pulse

TRUE or Corrected Statement

_____ 8. During the <u>secondary</u> survey, life–threatening conditions are identified and managed.

_____ 9. If a patient answers a question, it means that the <u>patient is oriented</u>.

_____ 10. If the patient is supine and has a blocked airway, <u>hyperextend the neck</u> to raise the tongue.

_____ 11. Control the cervical spine by manually maintaining the neck in a <u>neutral position</u>.

_____ 12. <u>Vital signs</u> should be checked before performing the head–to–toe secondary survey.

INTERPRETATION AND DOCUMENTATION

Completion

13. What is upper airway obstruction?

_____

_____

14. List at least two causes of hypovolemic shock.
    A. _____
    B. _____

15. List at least two findings that would help you recognize hypoxemia.

   A. _____

   B. _____

16. What is increased intracranial pressure?

   _____

   _____

17. List at least two causes of ventilatory failure.

   A. _____

   B. _____

TRUE or Corrected Statement

_____ 18. <u>Drooling</u> is a sign of air leakage into soft tissue.

_____ 19. Look and feel for dampness in dark clothing that may obscure <u>urinary incontinence</u>.

_____ 20. Hypoxemia and hypovolemic shock may cause a patient's <u>level of consciousness</u> to decrease.

_____ 21. A skull fracture should be suspected when the patient has <u>squirrel ears</u> or a Battle sign.

_____ 22. Blunt trauma that causes organ rupture and occult hemorrhage will cause abdominal <u>constriction and redness</u>.

Multiple Choice

23. Lethargy, increased pulse and respiratory rates, dyspnea, and cyanosis with pallor and mottling are signs most indicative of:

   A. hypovolemic shock.

   B. hypoxemia.

   C. septic shock.

   D. upper airway obstruction.

24. Trauma or disease that causes a headache is most often associated with:

   A. increased intracranial pressure.

   B. increased pulmonary hypertension.

   C. status asthmaticus.

   D. status epilepticus.

25. Which sign is most suggestive of a retroperitoneal hematoma?

   A. Bayline symptom

   B. Grey–Turner sign

   C. Hamman crunch

   D. Kehr position

26. Although a pediatric and adult assessment sequence is the same, which of the following factors require different intervention standards?
    A. Blood and fluid volumes
    B. Capillary refill responses
    C. Glasgow Coma Scores
    D. Intracranial pressure measurements

27. Dark vomitus, crushing chest pain, and throbbing eye pain are conditions that most likely suggest:
    A. early pregnancy.
    B. life–threatening conditions.
    C. onset of the flu.
    D. psychosomatic illness.

28. Delayed treatment can result in blindness in which condition?
    A. Conjunctivitis
    B. Astigmatic myopia
    C. Retinal detachment
    D. Transient ischemia

29. Why might a child require emergency intervention when an adult with the same injury would not need such care?
    A. A child's larynx is lower and posterior.
    B. A child's nasal passages are larger and wider.
    C. A child's tongue is relatively small and moveable.
    D. A child's trachea is narrower and more collapsible.

30. Which one of the following methods is best for summarizing clinical and numerical data?
    A. Checklists
    B. Flowsheets
    C. Narrations
    D. Photocopies

31. According to the Yale Observation Scales, which of the following crying characteristics is an ominous sign in an infant or young child?
    A. High–pitched cry
    B. No crying
    C. Sobbing tears
    D. Whimpering

2. Which one of the following statements is the best way to document a patient's living will or
   durable power of attorney for health care?
   A. Have the family complete standardized institutional forms.
   B. Keep entries of patient wishes in their medical record.
   C. Note advance directives in the SOAP charting format.
   D. Omit any reference to legal issues in the medical record.

Matching

	Condition		Child Characteristic
_____	33. Altered consciousness		A. Combative
_____	34. Early shock		B. Delayed capillary refill
_____	35. Increased intracranial pressure		C. Doughy skin texture
_____	36. Late shock		D. High–pitched cry
_____	37. Moderate dehydration		E. No tears
_____	38. Pai		F. Normal systolic pressure
_____	39. Respiratory distress		G. Rigid posturing
_____	40. Severe dehydration		H. Tripod positioning

Chapter 21

Recording Information

STUDY FOCUS

Patient records must be organized, accurate and concise. These notations must also be detailed enough to provide the readers with a complete picture of the patient's past, present and potential health care needs and interventions. Concentrate on developing your optimal record keeping skills.

LEARNING ACTIVITIES

GENERAL GUIDELINES

Completion

1. List four ways a patient's record enables you and your colleagues to care for a patient.

   A. _____

   B. _____

   C. _____

   D. _____

TRUE or Corrected Statement

_____ 2. Use an <u>outline form</u> to record the history and physical.

_____ 3. One way to record expected findings is to indicate the <u>absence of symptoms</u>.

_____ 4. Recording pain on a scale from 1 to 10 is an example of <u>objective</u> data.

_____ 5. The size of a lesion should be <u>compared to fruit or nuts</u>.

_____ 6. <u>Drawings</u> may be used to illustrate pain radiation.

_____ 7. Location of a finding may be recorded by using <u>clock positions</u>.

ORGANIZING AND ASSESSING DATA

Multiple Choice

8. The reasons why a person seeks health care as stated verbatim by the patient refers to the:
   A. chief complaint.
   B. past medical history.
   C. personal/social history.
   D. previous problem.

9. Which of the following information belongs in a family history?
   A. Chronic illnesses
   B. Current problems
   C. Hereditary diseases
   D. Personal data

10. Data relevant to a medical history includes:
   A. acute symptoms.
   B. chronic illnesses.
   C. cultural data.
   D. genetic risks.

11. Educational and economic information belongs in the:
    A. chief complaint history.
    B. family history.
    C. past medical history.
    D. personal/social history.

12. Objective data is usually recorded:
    A. along with the family history.
    B. by body systems and anatomic locations.
    C. in alphabetical order according to systems.
    D. with reference to subjective data.

13. The Tanner chart is used to record what type of data?
    A. Gestational age
    B. Language abilities
    C. Growth and development
    D. Level of self–care

14. When recording the history of older adults, you should:
    A. write the data as they were obtained.
    B. concentrate on the medical history.
    C. vary the growth and development section.
    D. follow the organized structure.

Matching

	Adult Findings	*Body Part or System*
_____	15. 4 + deep tendon reflexes	A. Abdomen
_____	16. Friction rub	B. Breasts
_____	17. Swollen joints	C. Cardiac
_____	18. Auricle alignment	D. Chest
_____	19. Hernia–scrotal	E. Ears
_____	20. Hemorrhoids	F. Eyes
_____	21. Thyroid tenderness	G. Female genitalia
_____	22. Facial symmetry	H. Head
_____	23. Bowel sounds	I. History data
_____	24. Nipple dimpling	J. Lymphatic
_____	25. Clubbing	K. Male genitalia
_____	26. Sinus swelling	L. Mouth and throat
_____	27. Homan sign	M. Musculoskeletal
_____	28. Consensual light response	N. Neck
_____	29. Uvula movement	O. Neurologic
_____	30. Murmur	P. Nose
_____	31. Retractions	Q. Peripheral vascular
_____	32. Discrete inguinal nodes	R. Rectum
_____	33. Uterine tenderness	S. Respiratory
_____	34. Hypertension	T. Skin

Infant Findings	Body Part or System

_____ 35. Hydrocele

_____ 36. Stridor

_____ 37. Lanugo

_____ 38. Tags or pits

_____ 39. Gestational age

_____ 40. Jitteriness

_____ 41. Umbilical redness

_____ 42. Cleft palate

_____ 43. Head position

_____ 44. Breast engorgement

_____ 45. Pilonidal dimple

_____ 46. Nasal flaring

_____ 47. Palmar creases

_____ 48. Cyanotic unless crying

_____ 49. Prominent labia

_____ 50. Red reflex

_____ 51. Bulging fontanels

A. Abdomen
B. Cardiac
C. Chest
D. Ears
E. Eyes
F. Female genitalia
G. Head
H. History data
I. Male genitalia
J. Mouth
K. Musculoskeletal
L. Neck
M. Neurologic
N. Nose
O. Rectum
P. Respiratory
Q. Skin

Completion

52. In the space provided, explain the process for determining problems and diagnoses.

_____

_____

_____

_____

_____

_____

PLANS AND RECORDS

Completion

53. List at least six things that are usually part of the proposed management plan.

A. _____

B. _____

C. _____

D. _____

E. _____

F. _____

54. What type of medical system is the SOAP note?

_____

_____

TRUE or Corrected Statement

_____ 55. A <u>genogram</u> can be used to document family history data.

_____ 56. Combined information about the thyroid gland, skin temperature, and estrogen use is usually noted as part of the <u>immunologic</u> history.

_____ 57. A stick person drawing is most useful for documenting pulse amplitudes and deep <u>organ palpation</u>.

_____ 58. Newborn history pertinent to a toddler's assessment belongs in the <u>past medical</u> section.

_____ 59. Symmetrical buttocks folds and palmar creases in infants is noted with other <u>neurologic</u> data.

_____ 60. The management plan is written after completing the <u>physical examination</u>.

PART II

Nursing Considerations and Nursing Diagnoses

INTRODUCTION

NURSING PROCESS

Nursing is both a science and an art, and as such, it is concerned with the physical, psychologic, sociologic, cultural, and spiritual concerns of the individual. To deal with the concerns, the nursing profession has developed a five-step process to provide an efficient method of organizing thought processes for clinical decision-making, problem solving, and the delivery of higher-quality and individualized patient care. The steps of nursing process are assessment, nursing diagnosis, planning, implementation, and evaluation. These steps are performed continuously throughout the patient's contact with the health care system and are the basis for all nursing actions in any setting. The nursing process combines all of the skills of critical thinking and creates a method of active problem-solving that is both dynamic and continuous. This process aids in determining what problems the individual has, which problems can be prevented, what kind and how much assistance is required, who can best provide such assistance, and what desired outcome is realistic. The process is goal directed and patient centered (depending on the setting, the patient may be an individual, a family, or a community).

Nursing today has seen a tremendous influx of new information and research. Due to this explosion of technology, nursing responsibilities have increased, thereby creating a greater need to expand and perfect assessment skills. The assessment phase of the nursing process is the foundation from which all future decisions will be based. It then goes without saying, that health care professionals today need a strong and in-depth background in assessment. Assessment begins with the first encounter with the patient and continues throughout the association.

To begin the process, the nurse obtains a comprehensive database. This data base has three components: (1) health history, (2) physical examination, and (3) diagnostic and laboratory tests. Together, these components provide the knowledge base for all decisions and actions. The data base grows as the nursing process progresses and changes as new data are revealed, the patient's condition changes, and the nurse-patient relationship grows. This approach is shared by all members of the health care team, and from this database, the health professionals make a judgment, or diagnosis, about the individual's health status.

The nurse obtains data from the patient in various ways, depending on the patient's condition, the nurse's abilities, and the type of information required. A judgment must be made as to which human need should be assessed first. Frequently an area of need is self evident and will determine the sequence of assessment. For example, anxiety, pain, dyspnea, and a lack of understanding can interfere with the nurse's ability to obtain a comprehensive database. Your patient's attention span and focus will be limited. These needs may require immediate intervention before completing the assessment phase. Flexibility is the key. Certain cognitive and emotional needs may take priority over your data collection. As the assessment process proceeds, these priorities will become evident.

The assessment phase begins with the health history and review of systems. Collecting appropriate data is the key to an accurate and comprehensive assessment. This process includes interview and observation. An individual's facial expressions, tone of voice, mannerisms, and nonverbal cues can provide information about the patient's emotional state, immediate comfort level, and general physical condition. The primary source of data, and often the best source, is the patient himself. Secondary sources include family members, friends, coworkers, or community service groups; these sources can be valuable as they supply alternative viewpoints to the patient's and add data unknown to the patient.

After establishing a rapport with the patient, the health care professional performs a physical examination to collect objective data. This then establishes a baseline for all assessment areas and is used to support information received during the interview. To obtain objective data, four techniques will be used: inspection, palpation, percussion, and auscultation.

The final component of the assessment phase is diagnostic and laboratory tests. In conjunction with a history and physical examination, these tests may confirm a diagnosis or provide valuable information about a patient's status and response to the therapy. It then becomes important for all health care providers to have a working knowledge and understanding of the information provided by diagnostic and laboratory testing.

This part of the Student Workbook was designed to supplement the textbook, *Mosby's Guide to Physical Examination* by Seidel, Ball, Dains, and Benedict. The textbook provides information concerning the first two phases of assessment, health history and physical examination. This supplement includes the third phase, as well, diagnostic and laboratory tests. It also addresses the second step of the nursing process, nursing diagnosis.

Each of the chapters in this supplement corresponds to a chapter in the textbook. Case studies and health promotion information are included at the end of the chapters.

GLOSSARY

Health assessment: the collection of data about an individual, family, or community using a holistic approach. Holistic health views the mind, body, and spirit as interdependent and functioning as a whole within the environment. The physical, psychological, sociological, cultural, and spiritual aspects are considered, as well as health perception and management, and stress and stress responses. The data base consists of subjective and objective information.

Physical assessment: the evaluation of the function of the body and functional abilities using subjective and objective data.

Physical examination: the examination of the body using the techniques of inspection, palpation, percussion, and auscultation. The database consists of objective data only.

Patient database: a pool of knowledge about the patient including the nursing history, physical examination, and results of diagnostic and laboratory tests.

Nursing process: a five-step process that provides an orderly, logical problem-solving approach for administering nursing care so that the patient's needs for such care are met comprehensively and effectively.

1. **Assessment**: the first phase of the nursing process; data are collected in a systematic process and provide the foundation for the remaining steps of the nursing process. It includes the gathering of information regarding the patient, the patient/family system, and/or the community.

2. **Nursing diagnosis**: analysis of data to identify the patient's problems and needs.

3. **Planning**: setting goals, identifying outcomes, and choosing interventions to create a plan of care to treat problems and needs identified in step 2.

4. **Implementation**: putting the plan into action.

5. **Evaluation**: determining the effectiveness of the plan and making changes if indicated.

Nursing diagnosis: an actual or potential patient health problem that a nurse is educationally prepared for and legally authorized to treat. The diagnoses used in this book are the approved labels developed by the North American Nursing Diagnoses Association (NANDA). They are a clinical judgment about an individual's, family's, or community's response to an actual or potential illness/condition. A nursing diagnosis provides the basis for the selection of nursing interventions to achieve outcomes for which the nurse is accountable.

Related factors (risk factors, etiology, identified causes, and/or contributing factors): the condition or situation that appears to demonstrate some type of patterned relationship with a specific nursing diagnosis. This forms the "related to" component of the patient diagnostic statement.

Defining characteristics (signs and symptoms): the abnormal or unexpected findings, both subjective and objective, that validate the selection of an actual nursing diagnosis.

Subjective data/findings: those statements by the patient concerning his/her thoughts and feelings. The nurse can not measure or directly observe these symptoms. The method of collection is through the interview process.

Objective data/findings: the data that are collected by the nurse using one or more of the senses (sight, smell, hearing, and touch). These signs are observable/measurable behaviors and physiologic functions of the patient. The data are collected through physical examination (inspection, palpation, percussion, and auscultation).

Sign: the objective or observable evidence or manifestation of a health problem.

Symptom: the subjectively perceptible change in the body or its functions that indicates disease or the phases of disease.

Growth and Measurement
(including Nutrition Assessment)

NURSING CONSIDERATIONS

The quality of a patient's life is affected by the quality and quantity of nutrients consumed and used. The body's nutritional status refers to the health of an individual as it is affected by the intake, storage, and use of nutrients. Proper nutrition promotes growth, maintains health, and helps the body resist infection and recover from disease or surgery.

Nutritional disorders can be seen in many settings and populations. Certain groups have a particularly high risk of developing nutritional deficiencies, such as those with low income, children, adolescents, pregnant or lactating women, and people over the age of 60. Malnutrition may be a primary disorder caused by insufficient nutrient intake or a secondary disorder caused by any condition that impairs digestion, absorption, or the use of nutrients.

Nurses are in an excellent position to recognize signs of poor nutrition and initiate interventions to facilitate change. Because food and fluid are basic biologic needs of all human beings, and the effects of malnutrition can be profound, it is important to make nutritional assessment a frequent part of your complete assessment throughout the association.

There are many conditions that place a patient at risk for nutritional problems, that is, stress, certain disease processes, hospitalization, surgery, and lifestyle habits. Even if your patient is not admitted with a nutritional problem, he still can be at risk within the hospital setting.

The effects of malnutrition can be devastating. During starvation, glycogen or carbohydrate stores are used first, but since these stores are small, they are usually exhausted within 15 to 20 hours. After that, caloric needs are supplied by conversion of skeletal muscle protein to glucose. As energy requirements continue, protein stores become severely depleted, which causes impaired wound healing, altered immune competence, and labored breathing. Continued starvation eventually leads to multiple organ failure and death. Malnutrition is associated with general debilitation, apathy, increased rates of morbidity and mortality, and greater medical expenses. The incidence and severity of malnutrition can be prevented or significantly reduced when it is identified and treated early.

Since prevention and early detection is the ultimate goal, a thorough nutritional assessment by the nurse becomes even more important. The components of a nutritional assessment include (1) health history, (2) physical examination, (3) anthropometry, and (4) laboratory data.

Health History
In addition to a general nursing history, the nurse obtains a more detailed diet history, food intake record, and psychosocial assessment to assess the patient's actual or potential nutritional needs. This information includes the patient's habitual intake of food and fluids, as well as preferences, allergies, problems, and other relevant areas.

Begin by asking the person to describe a typical day's diet, including fluids and snacks. A number of methods can be used to determine dietary intake, including the 24-hour diet recall, food frequency questionnaires, food diaries, and calorie counts. This information is then compared with established standards such as recommended daily allowances to make judgments about the adequacy or inadequacy of the diet.

There are many factors that influence diet that need to be taken into consideration. Such factors include preferences, dislikes, allergies, culture, habits, religion, and economics. Inquire about who purchases and prepares the food. Determine whether or not facilities for food storage and preparation are adequate.

Next, consider energy requirements by obtaining information about the person's activity level and medical history. The more active an individual is the more calories are required to support metabolism. Note any conditions that may deplete the body's energy stores by increasing the metabolic rate such as infection, trauma, surgery, burns, malignancies, and major wounds.

A number of factors are associated with or known to contribute to nutritional problems. Examples include persons receiving cancer therapy, poorly fitting dentures, medications and/or illnesses that cause a decreased appetite, nausea, pain, and sores in the mouth. Note the degree of stress, as well as the usual coping mechanisms.

Body image and relationships with others are frequently interrelated with food intake. For this reason it is important to assess the person's self-concept and social support patterns. Advertising promotes the idea that thinness and physical fitness are necessary to be happy and successful. Discuss with your patient whether he is happy with his weight and the way he looks. Does he like himself?

Physical Examination

The physical examination may reveal clinical signs that the history and laboratory data do not. Because improper nutrition affects all body systems, clues to malnutrition may be observed. It is important to remember that overt clinical signs of altered nutritional status occur late in the course of the problems and can have nonnutritional causes (see Table 4-16, p.112, in Seidel et al: *Mosby's Guide to Physical Examination*).

Physical assessment includes inspection, palpation, and anthropometry data. Begin by inspecting the patient's overall appearance. Pay particular attention to the skin, hair, mouth, eyes, nails, posture, muscles, extremities, and thyroid gland. The mouth includes the lips, teeth, gingivae, tongue and mucous membranes. Abnormalities in these areas may suggest a nutritional deficiency. Palpation, although less important than inspection for detecting nutritional deficiencies, can be used to detect enlarged glands (including the thyroid and parotid), liver, and spleen, which may indicate a nutrition-compromising disorder.

Anthropometry

Anthropometry is a system of measurement of the size and make-up of the body and specific body parts. Data includes height and weight, body frame size, skinfold evaluation, arm and arm muscle circumference, and in infants and children, head and chest size. These measurements provide information enabling the nurse to evaluate the height-weight relationships, which provides information related to under or over nutrition.

DIAGNOSTIC TESTS

Various laboratory studies are of particular value, since they are objective, can detect preclinical nutritional deficiencies, and confirm subjective findings. Keep in mind that abnormal findings may be caused by problems unrelated to nutrition.

Hemoglobin: measures the blood component that provides oxygen-carrying capacity; also used to detect iron deficiency anemia. With severe protein malnutrition, the hemoglobin level may reflect protein status.

Hematocrit: measures the percentage of red cells in total blood volume and iron status.

Serum lipids

Cholesterol: the main lipid associated with arteriosclerotic vascular disease. It can be found in muscles, red blood cells, and cell membranes, and is needed to form steroid hormones, bile acids, and most cell membranes. Most of the cholesterol we eat comes from foods of animal origin. Cholesterol is transported in the bloodstream by lipoproteins: high-density lipoproteins (HDL) and low-density lipoproteins (LDL). The HDLs (15%-35%) act as scavenger molecules facilitating removal of cholesterol from the body, while the LDLs (60%-75%) are associated with increased coronary heart disease.

Triglycerides: accounts for more than 90% of dietary intake and comprise 95% of the fat stored in tissues. This test is used to screen for hyperlipidemia and to determine the risk of coronary artery disease.

Transferrin test (total iron-binding capacity (TIBC) and serum iron): provides another parameter to assess visceral protein status. *Transferrin*, a protein and beta globulin, regulates iron absorption and transport in the body. This test evaluates iron metabolism in iron-deficiency anemia. Serum transferrin, with a half-life of 8 to 10 days, is an early indicator of visceral protein status. *Serum iron* refers to transferrin-bound iron, therefore, it measures the amount of iron bound to transferrin. *Iron-binding capacity* reflects the transferrin content of the serum and evaluates nutritional status.

Serum albumin: measures serum levels of albumin, which is a protein that is formed in the liver and helps maintain normal distribution of water in the body; approximately 52% to 60% of total protein is albumin; has a half-life of 17 to 20 days and is therefore not an early indicator of protein malnutrition.

Total protein: measures the protein content of the blood, aids in determining nutritional status, and indicates hyperproteinemia or hypoproteinemia.

Total lymphocyte count (TLC): along with skin antigen testing, TLC is used to measure immune function or the body's ability to fight disease; used to assess visceral protein status and cellular immune function.

Skin antigen tests: protein malnutrition is associated with impaired cell-mediated immunity; tests are used to assess immune function; commonly used antigens are *Candida albicans*, mumps, tetanus and purified protein derivative (PPD).

Nitrogen balance test: used to determine the patient's level of body protein breakdown; under normal conditions the body takes in through food and excretes in urine the same amount of protein each day. Nitrogen is released with the catabolism of amino acids and is excreted in the urine as urea. If the body is catabolizing more protein than it takes in, the body is in negative nitrogen balance. This imbalance occurs in cases of severe stress, injury, or disease. If negative nitrogen balance continues, the patient is at risk for developing protein malnutrition. Nitrogen balance studies involve calculating protein intake through dietary and/or intravenous means and measuring urine losses.

Creatinine height index (CHI): used to assess the amount of skeletal muscle mass. Creatinine is a protein, is a byproduct of muscle energy metabolism, and is produced at a rate depending on the muscle mass of the individual. It is constant as long as muscle mass remains constant. CHI calculates the amount of creatinine the body excretes over a 24-hour period and compares that value with ideal urinary creatinine from a standard table. A CHI of 60% to 90% of standard indicates moderate depletion; under 60% of standard indicates severe depletion.

NURSING DIAGNOSES
Altered nutrition: more than body requirements

Definition: the state in which the individual consumes more than adequate nutritional intake in relation to metabolic demands.

Related Factors

- Altered exercise pattern (lack of exercise, decreased exercise)
- Imbalance between activity level and caloric intake
- Excessive intake in relationship to metabolic need
    In response to stress or emotional trauma
    As a comfort measure/substitute gratification
    Learned eating behaviors
    Negative body image

Decreased self-esteem
Feelings of anxiety, depression, guilt, boredom, frustration
Perceived lack of control
- Decreased metabolic need
- Effects of drug therapy (appetite-stimulating)
- Ethnic and cultural values
- Lack of knowledge regarding nutritional needs

Defining Characteristics

Subjective: reported dysfunctional eating patterns, e.g., pairing food with other activities; concentrating food intake at end of day; eating in response to external cues such as time of day; eating in response to internal cues other than hunger, such as anxiety and reported sedentary level.

Objective: observed dysfunctional eating patterns (as noted in subjective); weight 10% to 20% over ideal for height and frame; triceps skinfold greater than 15 mm in men, 15 mm in women; measured food consumption exceeds American Dietetic Association recommendations for activity level, age, and sex.

Altered nutrition: less than body requirements

Definition: the state in which the individual consumes inadequate nutritional intake in relation to metabolic demands.

Related Factors

- Inability to ingest or digest food or absorb nutrients due to biologic, psychologic, or economic factors
    - Impaired absorption
    - Alteration in taste or smell
    - Dysphasia
    - Dyspnea
    - Stomatitis
    - Nausea and vomiting
    - Fatigue
    - Inability to chew
    - Decreased appetite
    - Decreased salivation
    - Effects of hyperanabolic or catabolic states (cancer, burns, infections, improper dieting)
    - Decreased level of consciousness
    - Stress
    - Decreased sense of taste/smell (due to effects of aging)
    - Knowledge deficit (lack of information, misinformation, misconceptions)

Defining Characteristics

Subjective: report loss of weight with adequate food intake; altered taste sensation; satiety immediately after ingesting food; abdominal pain with or without pathology; sore buccal cavity; abdominal cramping; diarrhea; lack of interest in food; aversion to eating; inadequate food intake less than recommended daily allowance; loss of hair.

Objective: body weight 20% or more less than ideal for height and frame; loss of weight with adequate food intake; inflamed buccal cavity; capillary fragility; diarrhea and/or steatorrhea; pale conjunctival and mucous membranes; poor muscle tone or skin turgor; loss of hair; decreased serum albumin and/or total protein; decreased serum transferrin and/or iron binding capacity; anemia; aversion to eating; food intake less than recommended daily allowance.

Related Nursing Diagnoses

Feeding self-care deficit
Fluid volume excess
Fluid volume deficit
Altered growth and development
Impaired tissue integrity
Altered oral mucous membrane
High risk for infection
Impaired swallowing

CASE STUDY

J.K., an 88-year-old widow, came to the physician's office for her yearly physical examination.

Health History

Chief complaint: " I feel fine except I'm tired all the time and have no appetite."

Present problem: for the last 6 to 7 months has been feeling increasingly tired; since she has not been able to drive due to poor eye sight for the past 8 months, it has been harder to obtain groceries; has little energy to cook; eats 1 to 2 meals per day; takes several naps throughout the day; sedentary lifestyle.

Past medical history: hypertension; arthritis.

Social history: lives alone in own home; approximate caloric intake/day is 600-800; neighbors will occasionally drive her to the grocery store; denies smoking or use of alcohol.

Physical Examination

General: 88-year-old thin female; ht 5'6", wt 97 lb; BP 178/96, pulse 110, resp 24, temp 98.8°F.

Inspection

Mouth: poorly fitting dentures; buccal mucosa is red and swollen; gingivae is red; lips are dry with angular lesions at corners of mouth; tongue is beefy red and swollen.

Eyes: pale conjunctivae, dry and dull.

Hair: dry, dull and thin.

Skin: dry, pale, several bruises noted on legs.

Nails: ridged and spoon-shaped.

Musculoskeletal: underdeveloped "wasted" appearance, bowlegs, prominent scapulas.

Palpation

Mouth: buccal mucosa and tongue tender to touch.

Hair: brittle.

Skin: generalized roughness, scaling noted on bilateral legs, poor turgor.

Nails: brittle.

Musculoskeletal: generalized poor tone, muscles soft and flaccid.

Gastrointestinal: liver 4 cm below costal margin and slightly tender.

Cardiovascular: heart rate 110, BP 178/96

Neurologic: decreased position and vibratory sense bilateral feet and hands with slight paresthesia.

Diagnostic Tests

Hemoglobin: 9 g/dl

Hematocrit: 22%

Red blood cells: 2.9 x 10^{12} cells/L

Lymphocytes: 15%

Serum iron: 59 g/dl

Transferrin: 200 mg/dl

Albumin: 2.0 g/dl

Total protein: 4 g/dl

Problems Identified for J.K.

Altered nutrition: less than body requirements related to anorexia and lack of access of groceries

Defining Characteristics

Subjective: states a decrease in appetite; verbalizes an increase in fatigue; verbalizes difficulties in obtaining groceries; complains of oral tenderness; eats 1 to 2 meals/day.

Objective: ht 5'6", wt 97 lb; pulse 110; BP 178/96; oral cavity is red and swollen; lips dry with angular lesions at corners of mouth; tongue beefy red and swollen; conjunctivae pale; eyes dry and dull; hair is dry, brittle and thin; skin is dry, rough, pale with scaling and bruises noted on both legs; poor skin turgor; generalized poor muscle tone with "wasted" appearance; prominent scapulas; muscles soft and flaccid; decreased position and vibratory sense bilateral feet and hands with slight paresthesia.

Activity intolerance related to generalized weakness

Defining Characteristics

Subjective: verbalizes fatigue, sedentary lifestyle, verbalizes little energy to cook.

Objective: "wasted" appearance, poor muscle tone, muscles soft and flaccid.

Altered oral mucous membranes related to malnutrition and poorly fitting dentures

Defining Characteristics

Subjective: verbalizes tenderness of buccal mucosa, fatigue.

Objective: poorly fitting dentures, buccal mucosa is red and swollen, gingivae is red, lips are dry with angular lesions at corners of mouth, tongue is beefy red and swollen.

Other Related Problems

Fatigue related to malnutrition

Fluid volume deficit related to inadequate replacement of fluid

Altered health maintenance related to inadequate support systems

High risk for infection related to malnutrition

Nursing Considerations and Nursing Diagnoses
to Accompany Chapter 5

Skin, Hair and Nails

NURSING CONSIDERATIONS

Health History

Assessment of the integumentary system begins with a complete health history, including information about the patient's skin, hair, and nails. It is important to remember that some skin disorders stem from other organ system problems and that all complaints, no matter how minor, should be considered. To decrease any anxieties that the patient may have, explain that questions about other parts of the body and general health are necessary to understanding the skin problem.

Physical Examination

The examination of the skin and appendages begins with a general inspection, followed by a detailed examination. Keep in mind that cultural and ethnic influences can predispose the patient to certain illnesses and may affect skin and mucous membrane coloring as well as hair texture and distribution. Ethnic backgrounds may influence dietary practices, rituals, and folk practices that may affect incidence, morbidity, and treatment of skin disorders. To do a complete assessment, the skin does need to be exposed. Be very careful to expose areas only as you need to see them and be aware of the patient's feelings. A comparison of symmetric anatomic areas is done throughout the examination. Use appropriate lighting; indirect natural daylight is preferred. There are several things to consider if you notice a color change in the patient's skin: (1) the lighting in the room, (2) the position of the patient or appendage, (3) the room temperature, (4) the patient's emotional status, (5) the cleanliness of the skin being assessed, and (6) the presence of edema. Through palpation note the texture, consistency, temperature, moisture, and elasticity. Always remember to wash your hands before and after touching a patient, and wear gloves when indicated since many skin conditions are contagious.

DIAGNOSTIC TESTS

A few of the most common diagnostic procedures to be included as a part of the total health assessment of a patient with skin, hair, or nail involvement are as follows.

Fungal examination: confirms the presence and identity of a fungal infection involving the skin and/or hair.

Skin cultures: confirm the presence, identity, and quantity of the organisms on the skin. There are several organisms present in low numbers on the healthy person's skin. When they multiply to excessive quantities, these same organisms may be pathogens.

Wound cultures: confirm the presence and identity of microorganisms within a wound.

Cutaneous immunofluorescence biopsy: aids in the diagnosis of certain disorders such as lupus erythematosis, blistering disease, and vasculitis. Skin biopsies are also used to confirm the histopathology of skin lesions to rule out other diagnoses and to follow the results of treatment.

NURSING DIAGNOSES

Impaired skin integrity: (actual or high risk for)
Definition: the state in which an individual experiences or is at risk for experiencing an alteration or disruption of the skin.

Related Factors

External (environmental)
- Hypothermia or hyperthermia
- Chemical substances on the skin
- Mechanical factors (shearing forces, pressure, restraint)
- Radiation

- Physical immobilization
- Excretions and secretions
- Humidity
- Insect/animal bites
- Trauma: injury/surgery
- Parasites

Internal (somatic)
- Altered nutritional state (obesity, maceration)
- Altered oxygen transport
- Altered sensation
- Autoimmune dysfunction
- Decreased circulation
- Altered pigmentation
- Edema

- Developmental factors (effects of aging)
- Effects of medications
- Infection
- Skeletal prominence
- Allergies (drugs, foods)
- Alterations in skin turgor (change in elasticity)
- Psychogenic

Defining Characteristics
Subjective: complains of itching, swelling, pain, numbness, of affected/surrounding area.
Objective: any disruption of skin surface; disruption of skin layers (incision, pressure sore); destruction of skin layers; invasion of body structures.
Examples: blisters, bruising, callus, chafing, cyanosis, denuded skin, dryness, erythema, induration, lesions, maceration, necrosis, pallor, pruritus

High risk for infection
Definition: the state in which an individual is at increased risk for being invaded by pathogenic organisms.

Risk Factors
- Inadequate primary defenses
  - Broken skin
  - Traumatized tissue
  - Decreased ciliary action
  - Stasis of body fluids
  - Change in pH of secretions
  - Altered peristalsis
- Inadequate secondary defenses
  - Decreased hemoglobin
  - Leukopenia
  - Suppressed inflammatory response
- Inadequate acquired immunity
- Malnutrition
- Pharmaceutical agents
- Trauma
- Invasive treatments/procedures
- Effects of chronic disease
- Tissue destruction
- Increased environmental exposure
- Insufficient knowledge to avoid exposure to pathogens

Impaired tissue integrity

Definition: the state in which an individual experiences damage to mucous membrane or corneal, integumentary, or subcutaneous tissue.

Related Factors
- Altered circulation
- Fluid deficit/fluid excess
- Impaired mobility
- Nutritional deficit/nutritional excess
- Knowledge deficit
- Irritants
  - Chemical (body excretions, body secretions, medications)
  - Mechanical (friction, pressure, shear)
  - Radiation (therapeutic radiation)
  - Thermal (temperature extremes)

Defining Characteristics

Damaged or destroyed tissue (cornea, mucous membrane, integumentary, subcutaneous)

Related Nursing Diagnoses

Pain
Body image disturbance
Altered nutrition: less than body requirements
Fluid volume deficit
Altered health maintenance
Hypothermia
Hyperthermia
Sensory/perceptual alteration (tactile)

CASE STUDY

Mr. K. is a 92-year old male who was admitted to the hospital from a long-term care facility with dehydration and coccyx decubitus ulcer.

Health History

Chief complaint: patient is confused.

Present problem: has had a decreased food/fluid intake for approximately 8 days; has an open lesion on coccyx present for approximately 3 weeks; treatment consisted of colloidal dressing changes every 8 hours; has been confused for approximately 2 years.

Past medical history: organic brain syndrome, hypertension.

Social history: patient is total care; activities include turning every 2 hours while in bed and up in chair 3 times per day for 2 hours; moans loudly whenever moved.

Physical Examination

General: 92-year-old thin male: ht 5'10"; wt 132 lb; BP 168/92, pulse 98, resp 22, temp 98.4°F.

Inspection

Skin: pale; reddened areas noted on both elbows and heels; lesion noted on coccyx 5 cm in diameter and 1 cm deep with small amount yellowish-green exudate; approximately 2 cm of redness noted around lesion; no peripheral edema noted.

Hair: thin; sparse; evenly distributed; dull; brittle; gray in color.

Nails: ridged; yellow in color.

Palpation:

Skin: warm; dry; scaly; loss of subcutaneous fat; bilateral radial and pedal pulses 1+; capillary refill >4 seconds; skin turgor poor.

Problems identified for Mr. K.

Impaired skin integrity related to mechanical factors such as pressure and physical immobilization.

Defining Characteristics

Objective: presence of lesion on coccyx; unable to turn self; confused and unable to care for self; resists movement, has reddened areas on both elbows and heels; decreased circulation to extremities; increased capillary refill; loss of subcutaneous fat; poor skin turgor; decreased nutritional status; effects of aging.

High risk for infection related to inadequate primary defenses (lesion on coccyx)

Defining Characteristics

Objective: **lesion on coccyx; poor overall circulation; capillary refill >4 seconds; poor skin turgor; decreased nutritional status.**

Other Related Problems

Altered nutrition: less than body requirements related to decreased level of consciousness.

Fluid volume deficit related to altered mental status.

Impaired tissue integrity related to altered circulation, nutritional deficit, and fluid deficit.

Self-care deficit: bathing/hygiene related to confusion.

Pain related to decubital ulcer.

HEALTH PROMOTION

Prevention/management of acne
- Keep hands and hair away from face
- Avoid constricting clothing over lesions
- Shampoo hair and scalp frequently
- Avoid exposure to oils and greases
- Eat a well-balance diet and avoid any foods that appear to cause skin flare-ups
- Keep skin clean: wash face 2-3 times daily
- Use a medicated soap or agent prescribed by physician
- Avoid vigorous rubbing of the skin
- Use cosmetics that are water-based rather tan cream-based
- Never leave cosmetics on face at night

Conditions that increase risk for skin cancer
- Light or fair complexion
- History of having bad sunburns or scars from previous burns
- Personal or family history of skin cancer
- Frequently work or play outdoors with exposure to the sun
- Exposure to x-rays or radiation
- Exposure to certain chemicals through work or hobby (coal, pitch, asphalt, petroleum)
- Repeated trauma or injury to any area resulting in scars
- Older than age 50
- Male gender
- Live in geographic location near the equator or at high altitudes

Ways to prevent skin cancer
- Avoid exposure to the sun
    - Wear long sleeves
    - Wear a hat to protect the face
- Avoid all sun lamps
- If exposure to the sun is unavoidable, use a sunscreen with a minimum sun protection factor (SPF) of 15

Teaching your patient how to recognize a potential problem
- Inspect your skin frequently; note all birthmarks, freckles, and moles
- Seek medical assistance if any of the following are noted:
    - Cange in color
    - Change in shape
    - Change in surface texture
    - Change in size
    - Change in the surrounding skin
    - A new mole
    - A sore that does not heal

Lymphatic System

NURSING CONSIDERATIONS

Health History

Unlike other body systems, the immune system and blood are not composed of simple organ groups. The immune system consists of billions of circulating cells and specialized structures, such as lymph nodes, that are located throughout the body. The blood includes plasma, blood cells and platelets that circulate throughout the body. Included in the defense against microorganisms are the spleen, tonsils, and adenoids. Whenever a patient reports symptoms such as frequent or recurring infections, slow wound healing, or blood clotting problems, the nurse should consider assessing the immune system and blood.

During the interview always remember to use terminology familiar to the patient, for example, bruising instead of "ecchymoses," swollen glands as opposed to "hypertrophy of lymphoid tissue," tired rather than "fatigue." The patient may report vague signs and symptoms with a gradual onset, which could indicate a disorder, simply be related to environmental or social stressors, or be attributed to aging. Signs and symptoms with a rapid onset usually indicate a disorder; those that begin insidiously or increase gradually may be related to hidden or chronic illness. It is important to remember that any change from the patient's usual status could be significant and requires investigation.

Obtain full biographic data, including age, sex, race, and ethnic background, because some immune and blood disorders occur more frequently in certain groups. Focus your questions on the more common signs and symptoms of immune and blood disorders: abnormal bleeding, swollen lymph nodes, fever, weakness, fatigue, and joint pain. Maintain a holistic approach in your health history because blood and immune system problems may result from problems in other body systems, may cause problems in other systems, or may impair other aspects of the patient's life.

Physical Examination

The superficial lymph nodes are dispersed throughout the body. Therefore, examination of the lymphatic system may be incorporated into the head-to-toe physical examination. If abnormalities of the lymph nodes or lymphatic vessels are suspect, you should examine the body areas that drain toward the affected lymph node or vessel for signs of inflammation, infection, swelling, or injury.

The superficial lymphatic system is examined by inspection and palpation. Enlarged lymph nodes are detected more easily by light palpation than by deep palpation. Be sure to palpate the entire area where a lymphatic chain may be located. Encourage the patient to report any tenderness experienced during the examination. Remember that small palpable lymph nodes are common and should be less than 1 cm wide, mobile, nontender, and discrete.

DIAGNOSTIC TESTS

Blood Studies

Complete blood cell count: determines the actual number of blood elements in relation to volume and quantifies abnormalities.

> **Erythrocytes (RBC)**: provides a count of the number of circulating RBCs in peripheral venous blood. An increase or decrease in the RBC count can provide clues to abnormalities such as anemia, hemorrhage, dehydration, and dietary deficiency.
>
> **Hematocrit (Hct)**: provides information concerning the percentage of RBCs and hydration status.
>
> **Hemoglobin (Hgb)**: serves as a vehicle for the transportation of oxygen and carbon dioxide and provides information concerning hydration status.

Red blood cell indices: provide information about the size (MCV), hemoglobin weight (MCH), and hemoglobin concentration (MCHC) of an average RBC and are helpful in classifying anemias.

> **Mean corpuscular volume (MCV)**: a measure of the average volume, or size of a single RBC.
>
> **Mean corpuscular hemoglobin (MCH)**: a measure of the average amount (weight) of hemoglobin within an RBC.
>
> **Mean corpuscular hemoglobin concentration (MCHC)**: a measure of the average concentration, or the percentage, of hemoglobin within a single RBC.

Leukocyte count (WBC): provides information concerning the number of leukocytes in periperhal venous blood.

Differential white cell count: evaluates WBC distribution and morphology, providing additional information about the body's ability to resist and overcome infection.

> **Neutrophils**: primary function is phagocytosis (killing and digestion of bacterial microorganisms); also reflect the body's reaction to inflammation.
>
> **Lymphocytes**: cells that migrate to areas of inflammation in both the early and late stages of inflammation; reflect the activity of antibody production; primary function is fighting chronic bacterial and acute viral infections.
>
> **Monocytes**: the body's second line of defense against infection; reflect phagocytic activity; capable of fighting bacteria in a way similar to the neutrophil, but they last longer in the bloodstream.
>
> **Eosinophils and basophils**: cells that play a role in the later stages of inflammation; are also active in allergic reactions; also can be stimulated by parasitic infections.

Erythrocyte sedimentation rate (ESR): used to detect inflammatory, neoplastic, infectious, and necrotic processes.

Platelet (thrombocyte) count: assesses the number of platelets in a blood sample; used to evaluate the number of platelets that are essential to blood clotting.

Partial thromboplastin time (PTT) (Activated partial thromboplastin time [APPT]): used to assess the intrinsic system and the common pathway of clot formation; evaluates all factors, except factors VII and XIII; Ptt is prolonged when any of these factors exist in deficient quantities.

Plasma thrombin time: estimates plasma fibrinogen levels by measuring the time needed for plasma to clot in the laboratory when thrombin is added; valuable test for detecting hypofibrinogenemia; may also be used to evaluate heparin therapy.

Plasma fibrinogen (factor I): measures the level of plasma protein fibrinogen available for coagulation.

Bleeding time (Duke and Ivy methods): measures the primary phase of hemostasis (the interactio of the platelet with the blood vessel wall and the formation of the homeostatic plug); one of th primary screening tests for coagulation disorders.

Direct Coombs test: used to detect autoantibodies against red blood cells that can cause cellula damage.

Indirect Coombs test: detects circulating antibodies against red blood cells; major purpose is to determine if the patient has serum antibodies to red blood cells that he or she is about to receive by blood transfusion.

Immunoelectrophoresis: identifies immunoglobulins IgG, IgA, and IgM in a serum sample; used to detect diseases of hypersensitivity, immune deficiencies, autoimmune diseases, chronic infections multiple myeloma, chronic viral infections, and intrauterine fetal infections.

Enzyme-linked immunosorbent assay (ELISA): identifies antibodies to bacteria, viruses, DNA and allergens, as well as substances such as carcinoembryonic antigens and immunoglobulins.

Skin tests: major reasons for skin testing are (1) to detect a person's sensitivity to allergens, such as dust and pollen, (2) to determine a person's sensitivity to microorganisms believed to cause disease. and (3) to determine whether a person's cell-mediated immune function is normal.

Types of skin tests:

1. Scratch tests: rows of small scratches are made on the patient's back or forearms and small quantities of allergens are introduced into these scratches.
2. Patch tests: a small piece of gauze is impregnated with the substance in question and applied to the skin of the forearm.
3. Intradermal tests: the substance that is being tested is introduced within the layers of the skin.

Examples of these skin tests are tuberculin skin test, Schick test, mumps test, blastomycosis test, and histoplasmosis test.

Radiologic Studies

Lymphangiography: used to examine the lymphatic channels and lymph nodes by injecting a radiopaque oil-based dye into the lymph vessels and obtaining radiographs immediately and again on the next day.

Computerized tomography: a noninvasive radiologic examination using computer-assisted x-ray study to evaluate the spleen, liver, or lymph nodes.

Magnetic resonance imaging (MRI): a noninvasive procedure providing images of soft tissue without the use of contrast dyes; used to evaluate such structures as the spleen, liver, and lymph nodes.

Radioisotope Studies

Scans: a radioactive isotope is injected intravenously and images from the radioactive emissions are used to evaluate different structures including the spleen, liver, bone, and bone marrow.

Biopsy Studies

Bone marrow: an invasive procedure involving the removal of bone marrow through a locally anesthetized site to evaluate the status of the blood-forming tissue.

Lymph node biopsy: an invasive procedure used to obtain lymph tissue for histologic examination to determine diagnosis and therapy.

NURSING DIAGNOSES

High risk for infection
Definition: the state in which an individual is at increased risk for being invaded by pathogenic organisms.

Risk Factors
- Inadequate primary defenses
  Broken skin
  Traumatized tissue
  Decreased ciliary action
  Stasis of body fluids
  Change in pH of secretions
  Altered peristalsis
- Inadequate secondary defenses
  Decreased hemoglobin
  Leukopenia
  Suppressed inflammatory response

- Inadaquate acquired immunity
- Malnutrition
- Pharmaceutical agents
- Trauma
- Invasive treatments/procedures
- Effects of chronic disease
- Tissue destruction
- Increased environmental exposure to pathogens
- Insufficient knowledge to avoid exposure to pathogens

Fatigue
Definition: the state in which an individual experiences an overwhelming sense of exhaustion and decreased capacity for physical and mental work.

Related Factors
- Decreased/increased metabolic energy production
- Increased energy requirements to perform activities of daily living
- Overwhelming physological or emotional demands

- Excessive social and/or role demands
- States of discomform
- Altered body chemistry: medications, drug withdrawal, chemotherapy

Defining Characteristics
Subjective: verbalization of an unremitting and overwhelming lack of energy; perceived need for additional energy to accomplish routine tasks; impaired ability to concentrate; decreased libido.
Objective: inability to maintain usual routines; increase in physical complaints, decreased performance; lethargy or listlessness; disinterest in surroundings/introspection; accident-prone.

Related Nursing Diagnoses
Activity intolerance
Altered nutrition: less than body requirements
Hyperthermia

CASE STUDY

R.L. is a 16-year-old female high school student admitted to the hospital with complaints of fever, sore throat, fatigue, and headache for approximately 1 week.

Health History

Chief complaint: fever, sore throat, fatigue, and headache.

Present problem: complaining of sore throat and headache for about 1 week; reports a lack of appetite and difficulty swallowing because of the sore throat; states she is so tired that all she wants to do is sleep; expresses concern about missing so much school.

Past medical history: measles, mumps, and chickenpox.

Family history: noncontributory.

Social history: nonsmoker.

Physical Examination

General: 16-year-old female: ht 5'4", wt 112 lb; BP 102/56, pulse 88, resp 20, temp 102.8°F.

Inspection

Throat: no tonsils, pharyngeal walls bright red with small amount of white exudate.

Abdomen: symmetrical, no edema noted.

Lymph nodes: no redness or edema noted in cervical, axillary, or groin area.

Palpation

Abdomen: no nodules palpated; complains of tenderness left upper quadrant; spleen 2 cm below costal margin.

Lymph nodes: enlarged anterior and posterior cervical nodes bilaterally, painful to palpation, 2 x 2 cm, firm, and mobile; anterior axillary nodes 2 x 2 cm bilaterally, painful to palpation, firm, and mobile; no enlargement noted in the groin area, nontender to palpation.

Diagnostic Tests

White blood cell count with differential: 20,000/mm^3; 55% are lymphocytes and monocytes; 20% are atypical lymphocytes.

Monospot test: positive for mononucleosis.

Throat culture: reveals beta-hemolytic streptococci.

Problems identified for R.L.

Activity intolerance related to fatigue from infectious process

Defining Characteristics:

Subjective: states she is so tired that all she wants to do is sleep; expresses concern about missing so much school because of the fatigue.

Objective: missing school.

Fatigue related to increased energy requirements related to infectious process

Defining Characteristics:

Subjective: verbalizes overwhelming lack of energy.

Objective: inability to maintain usual routines; missing school.

Altered nutrition: less than body requirements related to dysphagia

Defining Characteristics:

Subjective: reports anorexia and dysphagia

Objective: pharyngeal walls bright red with small amount white exudate; throat culture reveals beta-hemolytic streptococci.

Other Problems to Consider

Impaired swallowing related to dysphagia

Altered role performance related to fatigue

Altered sensory perception (gustatory) related to inflammation of oropharyngeal cavity

Hyperthermia related to infectious process

Pain (abdomen) related to infectious process

Altered oral mucous membranes related to infection

HEALTH PROMOTION

Methods of decreasing environmental inhalant antigens

- Avoid or minimize exposure to allergens

Animal dander

- Avoid fur-bearing pets, if possible
- Keep any family fur-bearing pet in outdoor enclosure
- Avoid feathers or kapok (pillows, mattresses, furniture)
- Avoid wool products (carpets, cloths, furniture, blankets)

Pollen spores

- Vacation in selected geographic ares, such as beach or sea, that are free of specific allergens during seasonal height
- Use air conditioning in home and in the car; keep windows closed in both home and car
- Limit time outdoors between sunset and sunrise, especially when windy
- Avoid going outside when pollen counts are high
- Avoid gardening, raking leaves, mowing lawn, or being near freshly cut grass
- Do not hang wash outside to dry (pollen and molds stick to wet wash)
- Minimize number of indoor plants (avoid dried plants)

Dust

- Use synthetic material, avoid wool and cotton (if must be used, wash frequently)
- Use a minimum of lint-producing articles
- Put away articles that are difficult to dust
- Daily damp dusting (no shaking of articles)
- Damp mop floors daily; vacuum frequently
- Avoid use of carpets and throw rugs, if possible
- Avoid use of overstuffed furniture, especially in the bedroom
- Use mattress and pillow encasements
- Use air conditioning as much as possible
- Use electrostatic air filter (clean filters every 2-3 weeks)
- Change/clean furnace filters every month

Head and Neck

NURSING CONSIDERATIONS

Health History

Because of the many structures involved in the head and neck, the nurse needs to organize the health history to elicit information on a wide range of topics. Begin by investigating the patient's current, past, and family health status.

Headaches are probably the most common type of pain experienced by human beings. The majority are classified as functional headaches of benign vascular or muscle-contraction origin, whereas the remainder are organic headaches caused by intracranial or extracranial disease. Chronic headache of benign origin is not only the most common, but also may be the least effectively treated physical disorder. Symptoms are often vague, signs are difficult to pinpoint, and timing and frequency may vary. A careful and complete history can help sort out these vague but important variables. It may also be helpful to have the patient keep a diary of headache episodes with specific details to aid in determining the type of headache, as well as the precipitating events.

Assessment of the endocrine system can be difficult and requires excellent clinical skills to detect manifestations of disorders. Hormones affect every body tissue and system, causing diversity in the signs and symptoms of endocrine dysfunction. The manifestations of a dysfunction may be nonspecific or very specific, thus requiring keen skills to identify the disorder. Assessment begins with a detailed and careful history to help sort out the possible causes. Some signs of an endocrine dysfunction are specific, and therefore it is easier to identify the cause, such as exophthalmos in hyperthyroidism. It is the nonspecific signs that make diagnosis more difficult. These signs include fatigue, depression, altered sleep patterns, changes in energy level, alterations in mood and/or weight, and changes in sexual function.

Pay specific attention to growth and development patterns, weight distribution and changes, and compare these factors with the normal findings. When comparing height in patients, make sure the charts are race specific because significant racial differences exist in children and adults.

Include questions about the general state of health and whether there have been any changes. Note whether any problem has affected the patient's ability to function at work, at home, or in society. Inquire about previous hospitalizations and surgeries, and any medications. Since heredity can play a major role in the cause of endocrine problems, it is important to include a family history. Stressors of any kind can affect the endocrine system. Consider the patient's place of employment, kind of work, ability to meet job requirements, and the amount of stress involved. Inquire about finances and marital status, since they often are causes of stress. Note previous and present coping patterns and discuss family support.

If an endocrine problem is suspected, the nurse should investigate all body systems because of the systemic effects of hormones. A complete review of systems can provide valuable additional information that may lead to a specific dysfunction.

Physical Examination

Begin the examination by noting the patient's general appearance, including physical growth and development, level of consciousness and orientation, and appearance and appropriateness of dress. Since an endocrine dysfunction can affect the development and maturation of the body, it is important to assess the head, face, and neck for size, shape, contour, color, and symmetry. Keep in mind that certain structures and facial features are characteristic of race, such as the prominent epicanthal folds in Asians. Throughout the entire examination note the patient's spontaneous facial expression because this can be a clue to the patient's psychologic state, or it can reveal physical distressor pain.

DIAGNOSTIC TESTS

Thyroid

Calcitonin: used to aid in the diagnosis of cancer of the thyroid; levels will be increased in medullary carcinoma, occasionally in patients with other tumors, and in some instances of renal failure.

Thyroid-stimulating hormone (TSH): TSH is produced by the anterior pituitary gland and causes the release and distribution of stored thyroid hormones. This test is used to diagnosis primary hypothyroidism and to differentiate primary form secondary hypothyroidism by determining the actual circulatory level of TSH.

Thyrotropin-releasing hormone (TRH) stimulation test: done to assess the responsiveness of the anterior pituitary gland and to differentiate among the three types of hypothyroidism: primary, secondary, and tertiary. When TRH is injected, a rise in TSH indicates that the pituitary gland is functioning.

Thyroxine-binding globulin (TBG): measures the levels of TBG, which is helpful in determining the amount of bound and active T3 and T4.

Thyroxine T4: used in the evaluation of thyroid function by a direct measurement of the concentration of T4 in the blood serum; commonly done to rule out hyperthyroidism and hypothyroidism.

Triiodothyronine (T3) by radioimmunoassay (T3-RIA): a quantitative determination of the total T3 concentration in the blood; the test of choice in the diagnosis of T3 thryotoxicosis.

Triiodothyronine uptake (T3 resin uptake): an indirect measurement of the unsaturated thyroxine-binding globulin in the blood; useful for the diagnosis of hypothyroidism or hyperthyroidism.

Thyroid scan: measures the uptake of radioactive iodine by the thyroid; used for the evaluation of thyroid size, position, and function.

Thyroid ultrasound: used to determine the size of the thyroid, to differentiate cysts from tumors, and to reveal the depth and dimension of thyroid goiters and nodules.

Head

X-ray (skull): x-rays allow the visualization of the bones and nasal sinuses to identify fractures, tumors, vascular abnormalities, and cranial anomalies.

Computed tomography (CT): the use of radiologic imaging and computer analysis; provides a three-dimensional view of the brain and spinal cord; aids in the detection and evaluation of tumors, trauma, abscesses, hemorrhages, and abnormal brain development.

Magnetic resonance imaging (MRI): provides images of body tissues; used in the evaluation of cerebral infarctions, tumors, central nervous system (CNS) disorders such as congenital anomalies, and the condition of blood vessels and determining blood flow.

NURSING DIAGNOSES

Pain

Definition: the state in which an individual experiences and reports the presence of severe discomfort or an uncomfortable sensation.

Related Factors

- Inflammatory process
- Muscle spasm
- Effects of trauma/surgery
- Immobility-Pressure
- Infectious process
- Overactivity
- Ischemia
- Injuring agents (biologic, chemical, physical, psychologic)

Defining Characteristics

Subjective: verbal reports of pain, discomfort, anxiety, uncomfortable sensation.

Objective: guarding, limping, facial mask or grimace, increased respirations, increased heart rate, increased blood pressure, anxious, restlessness, nausea, vomiting, diaphoresis, moaning, crying, pacing, self focusing.

Chronic pain

Definition: the state in which an individual experiences pain that continues for longer than 6 months.

Related Factors

- Effects of chronic or terminal illness
- Muscle spasm
- Inflammation
- Chronic psychosocial disability

Defining Characteristics

Subjective: verbal report of pain, fear of reinjury, altered ability to continue previous activities, changes in sleep patterns, preoccupation with pain.

Objective: facial masks of pain, anorexia, weight loss, insomnia, guarded movement, depression, personality changes, irritability.

Ineffective individual coping

Definition: the state in which an individual demonstrates impaired adaptive behaviors and problem-solving abilities.

Related Factors

- Situational crises
- Maturational crises
- Personal vulnerability
- Inadequate coping skills
- Unrealistic perceptions
- Multiple stressors/life changes
- Major changes in lifestyle
- Inadequate relaxation/leisure activities
- Low self-esteem

- Unmet expectations
- Poor nutrition
- Work overload
- Too many deadlines
- Unrealistic perceptions
- Inadequate support systems
- Little or no exercise
- Knowledge deficit regarding

(therapeutic regimen, disease process, prognosis)
- Sensory overload
- Severe pain
- Overwhelming threat to self
- Impairment to nervous system

Defining Characteristics
Subjective: verbal reports of inability to cope; inability to meet expectations; inability to ask for help; inability to problem solve; verbal manipulation, reports of chronic worry/anxiety/depression; lack of appetite; chronic fatigue; insomnia; general irritability.
Objective: insomnia; physical inactivity; substance abuse; alteration in societal participation; destructive behavior toward self or others; inappropriate use of defense mechanisms; change in usual communication patterns; inability to meet or take responsibility for basic needs; exaggerated fear of pain, death; general irritability; high rate of accidents or illnesses; frequent headaches/neckaches; indecisiveness; overeating; excessive smoking; excessive drinking; irritable bowel; poor self-esteem; lack of assertive behaviors.

Sleep pattern disturbance
Definition: the state in which an individual experiences disruption of the quality or quantity of sleep patterns, which causes discomfort.

Related Factors
- Effects of pregnancy
- Side effects of medications
- Pain
- Inactivity
- Diarrhea
- Urinary frequency
- Incontinence
- Nausea
- Lifestyle disruptions
- Demands of caring for others
- Stress
- Fear or anxiety
- Depression
- Nightmares
- Sensory overload
- Unfamiliar environment
- Circadian rhythm disturbances (shift work)

Defining Characteristics
Subjective: verbal reports of difficulty falling asleep, restlessness, frequent awakening, napping during day, difficulty in concentration, reports not feeling rested, awakening earlier or later than desired.
Objective: headache, dark circles under eyes or reddened eyes, lethargy, restlessness, listlessness, disorientation, increasing irritability, napping during day, remaining asleep, mood alterations, difficulty in concentration, frequent yawning, hand tremors, ptosis of eyelid, expressionless face, changes in posture, thick speech with mispronunciation and incorrect words.

CASE STUDY

L.B.. is a 30-year-old single mother who seeks medical attention for complaints of nervousness, ir to sleep, and neck discomfort.

Health History

Chief complaint: complains of nervousness, inability to sleep and neck discomfort.

Present problem: for approximately 1 month has become increasingly more tired but with an inability t complains of being restless, nervous and sometimes shaky; reports crying frequently, being exceptionally b by the summer heat, and intolerant of loud noises; has lost 15 lb in the last month but reports always being hun eating frequently throughout the day.

Past medical history: mumps and measles, age 6; broken right arm, age 12.

Family history: mother died of heart attack, age 57; father alive and well.

Social history: divorced 5 months ago; single parent of 3-year-old girl and 5-year-old boy; working full ti secretary for a law firm; verbalizes that for the last month has been very tired and that it is hard to care for the c and work; states she receives no family support and is concerned about who will care for the children if she

Physical Examination

General: 30-year-old female: ht 5'6", wt 117 lb; BP 140/60, pulse 134, resp 24, temp 99.0°F.

Inspection: skin pink with perspiration present; quick muscle response to sudden noise noted; fine tremors hands; diffuse visible enlargement of anterior aspect of neck.

Palpation: skin warm to touch; bilateral biceps and patellar reflexes 4+; thyroid: no nodules, firm but pliabl in width, rises symmetrically with swallowing, tender to palpation; supraclavicular and infraclavicular lympt approximately 2cm, soft, movable, tender to palpation.

Diagnostic Tests

Thyroxine (T4) and triiodothyronine (T3): levels elevated.

Thyroid scan: shows enlargement of the thyroid.

Electrocardiogram: shows sinus tachycardia, rate 134.

Problems identified for L.B.

Pain related to inflammatory process
Defining Characteristics
Subjective: complains of tenderness during palpation of thyroid and clavicular lymph nodes.
Objective: enlarged thyroid and lymph nodes.

Altered nutrition: less than body requirements related to increased metabolic need
Defining Characteristics
Subjective: reports always being hungry and eating frequently throughout the day.
Objective: lost 15 lb in 1 month; T3 and T4 levels increased.

Hyperthermia related to increased heat production greater than dissipation.
Defining characteristics
Subjective: reports being exceptionally bothered by the summerheat.
Objective: skin warm with perspiration present; temperature 99.0°F.

Sleep pattern disturbance related to increased metabolic rate and restlessness

Defining Characteristics

Subjective: complains of fatigue but with an inability to sleep.

Objective: restlessness; irritability; T3 and T4 levels increased.

Other Related Problems

Ineffective individual coping related to hypersensitivity to environmental stimuli

Activity intolerance related to fatigue

High risk for decreased cardiac output related to increased sympathetic stimulation

Anxiety related to change in health status and role functioning

HEALTH PROMOTION

Interventions for persons with headaches

- Promote rest and relaxation
  - Relaxation techniques, including biofeedback
  - Diversional activity
  - Regular sleeping patterns
  - Regular physical exercise
  - Provision for periodic rest periods
  - Heat applied to base of neck to relax tense muscles
  - Listen to soft, relaxing music
- Promote comfort
  - Quiet, peaceful environment
  - Rest in darkened room with minimal sensory stimulation
  - Cold packs to forehead or base of head
  - Pressure applied to temporal artery area
  - Judicious use of medication

Eyes

NURSING CONSIDERATIONS

Health History

Begin the interview by asking about the patient's current eye health status. If there are no complaints in this area, ask more general history questions about the eye. In the case of a specific complaint, obtain a complete description of the problem and any others. The existence of a problem with vision should lead to other questions in the area of self-care abilities and the potential for injury. Determine the date of the last eye examination and the patient's adherence to a recommended schedule of eye and vision examinations. Note whether the person wears contact lenses or glasses and include information concerning the care and cleaning of these items. Include information about eyestrain and headaches, which would indicate a problem with vision. Finally, note any pathologic conditions that could affect the eyes and vision, such as cataracts, glaucoma, hypertension, diabetes and infection.

Physical Examination

Assessment of the eye includes evaluating the internal and external structures of the eye and testing the patient's vision. Inspection and palpation are used; however, inspection is the predominant technique used to assess the eye. Perform the examination in a room that is well-lit, but one where you can control the amount of light.

DIAGNOSTIC TESTS

Electro-oculography (EOG): used in the study of suspected and acquired degeneration of the retina; helpful in evaluating the functional state of retinal pigment epithelium, as in retinitis pigmentosa.

Electroretinography (ERG): also used to study hereditary and acquired disorders of the retina, including partial and total color blindness, night blindness, retinal degeneration, and detachment of the retina.

Echogram of the eye: helpful in the removal of foreign bodies and allows for the study of the posterior parts of the eye; can also be used in evaluating retinal detachment.

Eye and orbit sonograms: used to describe both normal and abnormal tissues of the eye when no alternative visualization is possible because of opacities. The information is used in the management of eyes with large corneal leukomas or conjunctival flaps and in the evaluation of eyes for keratoprosthesis.

Tonometry (Schiotz and Applanation tonometer): used to measure the intraocular pressure of the eye and aids in the diagnosis of glaucoma.

NURSING DIAGNOSES

Sensory/perceptual alteration (visual)

Definition: The state in which an individual experiences an interruption or change in reception and/or interpretation of stimuli by receptors for sight.

Related Factors

- Effects of:
  Aging
  Stress
  Congenital or hereditary disorder
  Neurologic impairment (disease, trauma, or defect)
- Restriction of head/neck motion

- Failure to use protective eye devices
- Improper use of contact lens
- Difficulty in adjustment to corrective lens
- Persistent visual stimulation

Defining characteristics

Subjective: verbal reports of headache, blurring, spots, double vision, difficult seeing near and/or distant objects, photosensitivity.

Objective: excessive tearing, inflammation, lack of blink or corneal reflex, squinting, holding objects too close or at a distance for viewing, colliding with objects, abnormal results of vision testing.

Diversional activity deficit

Definition: the state in which an individual experiences reluctance or inability to participate in activities that pass the time or provide distraction or gratification.

Related Factors

- Effects of chronic illness
- Frequent lengthy treatments
- Unwillingness to learn new skills or acquire new interests
- Social isolation

- Confined to bedrest
- Preoccupation with job
- Decreased economic resources

Defining characteristics

Subjective: verbal reports of boredom, a desire for activity or work, an inability to participate in usual hobbies because of physical limitations or hospitalization.

Objective: weight loss or gain, yawning, crying, restlessness; preoccupation with self, napping during day, apathy or hostility, lethargy, withdrawn.

Impaired home maintenance management

Definition: the state in which an individual experiences the inability to independently maintain a safe, growth-producing immediate environment for self or others.

Related Factors

- Impaired mental status
- Substance abuse
- Effects of chronic debilitating disease
- Depression
- Lack of knowledge
- Lack of motivation
- Decreased financial resources
- Insufficient family organization or planning
- Inadequate support systems
- Unfamiliarity with neighborhood resources

Defining characteristics

Subjective: household members verbalize difficulty in maintaining their home in a comfortable fashion, outstanding debts or financial crises, requests for assistance with home maintenance.

Objective: accumulation of dirt, food, or hygienic wastes; unwashed or unavailable cooking equipment, clothes, or linen; family members anxious and/or exhausted; repeated hygienic disorders, infestations, or infections; disorderly surroundings; inappropriate household temperature; lack of necessary equipment or aids; presence of vermin or rodents; offensive odors.

Self care deficit: bathing/hygiene/dressing/grooming/ feeding/toileting

Definition: the state in which an individual experiences impaired ability independently to: (___).

Related Factors

- Neuromuscular impairment
- Musculoskeletal impairment
- Cognitive impairment
- Sensory impairment
- Trauma
- Surgical procedures
- Restrictive devices
- Imposed restrictions
- Activity intolerance
- Pain/discomfort
- Ineffective coping with body change
- Depression
- Severe anxiety

Defining characteristics

Subjective: verbal reports of difficulty performing daily activities.

Objective: partial or complete inability in performing desired activities.

Related Nursing Diagnoses

Altered role performance
Social isolation
Impaired social interaction
Impaired adjustment

Ineffective individual coping
Personal identity disturbance
High risk for injury

CASE STUDY

J.M. is a 53-year-old female who sought medical attention with complaints of headaches and difficulty seeing objects from the side.

Health History

Chief complaint: frequent headaches and difficulty seeing objects to the side.

Present problem: for approximately 3 weeks has been having an increase in frequency of headaches; also states that she has more difficulty seeing objects from the side; states that she sees halos around bright lights; states the halos and headaches make it hard to do her needlepoint.

Past medical history: insulin dependent diabetes for approx. 15 years (takes 15U Reg and 5U NPH insulin every AM with 5U Reg insulin around 5PM), hospitalized several times for control of diabetes; hypertension for approx. 4 years (controlled with medication).

Family history: mother: died age 67 with a myocardial infarction; had diabetes and glaucoma; father: died at age 45, history unknown.

Social history: nonsmoker; denies alcohol use; last eye exam 5 years ago; wears glasses; states does not check her glucose level regularly, just when she feels bad, because it is too expensive; reports that she sometimes skips taking her insulin when she feels good.

Physical Examination

General: 53-year-old female: ht 5'7", wt 157 lb; BP 146/86, pulse 76, resp 20, temp 98.2 F.

Visual acuity: right eye: 20/40; left eye: 20/50; ne.

Visual fields: decreased bilaterally, in all directions.

Extraocular muscles: movement intact bilaterally; corneal light reflex symmetrical; no nystagmus.

External eye: palpebral fissures--equal; brows, lids and lashes--evenly distributed; conjunctiva--pink without discharge; sclera--white, few small blood vessels noted at cornices; cornea--clear, arcus senilis present; lacrimal apparatus--no excessive tearing, no regurgitation of material from lacrimal sac; pupils--equal, round, react to light, and accommodate.

Ophthalmic examination: full red reflex present bilaterally; AV ratio 2:5; optic disc round, light gray with marked glaucomatous cupping; shallow anterior chamber; retina shows several small exudates on macula bilaterally.

Diagnostic Tests

Tonometry: reveals an increase in intraocular pressure (24 mm Hg).

Blood glucose: per glucometer = 275 mg/dl.

Problems identified for J.M.

Sensory/perceptual alterations (visual) related to increased ocular pressure, decreased peripheral vision and funduscopic abnormalities.

Defining Characteristics

Subjective: complaints of headache, difficulty seeing objects from the side, seeing halos around bright lights.

Objective: decreased peripheral vision, funduscopic abnormalities, increased intraocular pressure.

Diversional activity deficit related to visual defects and headaches

Defining Characteristics

Subjective: complains of difficulty seeing objects from the side, sees halos around bright lights, states that the halos and headaches make it hard to do her needlepoint.

Objective: decreased peripheral vision, funduscopic abnormalities, increased intraocular pressure.

Knowledge deficit related to relationship between vision changes and diabetes

Defining Characteristics

Subjective: reports she does not test her glucose level regularly; she sometimes skips taking her insulin when she is feeling good.

Objective: last eye examination was 5 years ago; present glucose level = 275 mg/dl.

HEALTH PROMOTION

Care of healthy eyes

- Avoid placing anything in the eye including your fingers
- Utilize good hand washing technique before and after contact with the eyes
- Discard any opthalmic solution that is cloudy, discolored, has been opened for 3 months or more, or contains particles
- Use good lighting when reading and doing work that requires careful visual focus
- Provide periodic rest periods when doing extremely fine work
- Discard mascara after 3 months
- Avoid self-treatment of eyes, seek medical attention when a problem arises
- All persons over the age of 40 should have regular screening for glaucoma

Preventing eye injuries

- Prevention of unintentional injury to the eyes should be stressed in child and adult education (e.g., care in theuse of BB guns, slingshots, water guns)
- Use protective goggles and/or break-resistant corrective lenses when engaging in active sports and selected occupations (e.g., seat belts and shoulder harnesses in cars; goggles and helmets while riding bikes)
- Use of protective goggles or special dark glasses to protect eyes from prolonged exposure to very bright light such as sunlight
- Use special protection from sudden flashes of light, chemicals and/or heat that occur in some industrial occupations

Nursing Considerations and Nursing Diagnoses
to Accompany Chapter 9
Ears, Nose, and Throat

NURSING CONSIDERATIONS
Health History
Many problems related to the ear are a result of childhood illnesses and/or from problems of adjacent organs. Therefore, it is necessary to obtain a careful and complete assessment of past medical problems. Acute or chronic problems such as otitis media, perforations of the eardrum, drainage, mumps, and/or measles, in childhood or adulthood, need to be discussed and recorded. Information about allergies and sinus problems is also important to obtain because the eustachian tube can become edematous and prevent aeration of the middle ear, which may effect hearing. Pregnant women and women of childbearing age should be questioned regarding whether they were vaccinated against rubella or ever had rubella. Congenital hearing losses can result from rubella or influenza in the first trimester of pregnancy. Discuss and record any previous hospitalizations involving trauma and/or surgeries involving the ear, tonsils, adenoids, or sinuses. Information about past and current medications that can produce hearing loss, tinnitus, and disequilibrium should be obtained. Examples of such medications are aminoglycosides, salicylates, antiprotozoal agents, and analgesics.

Another area of importance is the patient's social and personal history. Discuss and obtain information concerning the patient's oral and ear care patterns, nutrition, and smoking history. The patient should be questioned regarding type of employment or exposure to environments that have excessive noise levels, such as working with machinery, listening to amplified music, and firing of firearms.

Physical Examination
The examination of the nose, mouth, and throat provides the opportunity to inspect, directly or indirectly, parts of the upper respiratory system and the first part of the digestive system. It is, therefore, an important part of every physical examination.

The body's gastrointestinal tract begins with the oral cavity, including such structures as the lips, salivary glands, tongue and taste buds, gingiva, teeth, hard and soft palates, uvula, tonsils, and pharynx. Any problems with these structures could cause an alteration in digestion and the nutritional status of the patient.

Air, which is inhaled through the nose is warmed, humidified, and filtered before entering the trachea. Common problems associated with the nose include trauma, obstruction, and irritation or drainage secondary to colds and allergies. Depending on the part of the country in which the patient resides, allergies and sinus problems can be prevalent.

The assessment of the ear includes the external, middle, and inner structures, the hearing pathway, and equilibrium. Problems with any of these structures can cause hearing impairment. The health history interview provides a good opportunity to collect objective data regarding the patient's ability to hear. Clues such as posturing of the head and appropriateness of responses should be noted.

DIAGNOSTIC TESTS

Audiometry: useful as a screening test for hearing acuity and as a diagnostic test for determining the degree and type of hearing loss.

Culture and sensitivity: cultures may be taken from the ears, nose, sinuses, mouth and throat to diagnose bacterial infections. Sensitivities may be done on the cultures to aid in the selection of effective antibiotic therapy.

NURSING DIAGNOSES

Sensory/perceptual alteration (auditory, kinesthetic, gustatory, tactile, olfactory)

Definition: the state in which an individual experiences an interruption or change in reception and/or interpretation of stimuli by receptors for sight, hearing, body position, taste, touch, or smell.

Related Factors
- Chemical alterations
  Endogenous (electrolyte imbalance, elevated blood-urea nitrogen, elevated ammonia, hypoxia)
  Exogenous (central nervous system stimulants or depressants, mind-altering drugs)
- Altered environmental stimuli, excessive or insufficient
  Therapeutically restricted environment (isolation, intensivecare, bed rest, traction, incubator, confining illnesses)
  Socially restricted environment (institutionalization, home-bound, aging, chronic illness, dying, infant deprivation, bereaved, stigmatized, mentally ill, mentally retarded, or mentally handicapped)
- Altered sensory reception, transmission and/or integration
  Neurologic disease, trauma, or deficit
  Altered status of sense organs
  Inability to communicate, understand, speak, or respond
  Sleep deprivation
  Pain

Defining Characteristics
Subjective: verbal reports of anxiety, fatigue, indication of body image alteration, reported change in sensory acuity (photosensitivity, hypo/hyper peresthesias, diminished/altered sense of taste), pain, fear.

Objective: change in muscle tension; fatigue; measured change in sensory acuity; change in problem-solving abilities (lack or/poor concentration); alteration in posture; exaggerated emotional responses, rapid mood swings; change in behavior pattern; apathy; restlessness; irritability; anger; depression; inappropriate responses; hallucinations; disordered thought sequence; bizarre thinking; daydreaming; noncompliance, altered conceptualization; altered communication patterns, change in usual response to stimuli; altered abstraction; disoriented to time, place, or person.

Sensory/perceptual alteration (auditory)
Related Factors
- Effects of aging
- Neurologic impairment
- Effects of certain antibiotics
- Excessive ear wax, fluid, or foreign body in ear
- Social isolation
- Stress
- Failure to use protective ear devices
- Continuous exposure to excessive noise
- Psychoses

Defining Characteristics
Subjective: verbal reports of tinnitus.
Objective: abnormal hearing test; lack of startle reflex; failure to respond to verbal stimuli; cupping of ears; inattentiveness; withdrawal; daydreaming; auditory hallucinations; inappropriate responses; delayed speech or language development.

Sensory/perceptual alteration (kinesthetic)
Related Factors
- Effects of inner ear inflammation
- Neurologic impairment
- Side effects of tranquilizers, sedatives, muscle relaxants, or antihistamines
- Sleep deprivation

Defining Characteristics
Subjective: verbal reports of nausea, vertigo, motion sickness.
Objective: falling, stumbling, motor incoordination, alteration in posture, inability to sit or stand.

Sensory/perceptual alteration (gustatory)
Related Factors
- Inflammation of nasal mucosa
- Side effects of certain medications
- Aging
- Effects of trauma
- Neurologic impairment

Defining Characteristics
Subjective: verbal reports of decreased sensitivity to tastes; decreased appetite.
Objective: increased use of seasoning.

Sensory/perceptual alteration (olfactory)
Related Factors
- Inflammation of nasal mucosa
- Foreign body in nasal passage
- Effects of aging
- Neurologic impairment

Defining Characteristics
Subjective: verbal reports of decreased sensitivity to smells, decreased appetite.
Objective: unable to detect various odors.

Altered oral mucous membrane

Definition: the state in which an individual experiences alteration of the integrity of the oral cavity.

Related Factors
- Dehydration
- Effects of chemotherapy, medication, and radiation to head/neck
- Immunosuppression
- Inadequate oral hygiene
- Infection
- Mouth breathing
- Malnutrition/vitamin deficiency
- NPO status for more than 24 hours
- Chemical trauma (e.g., acidic foods, alcohol, drugs, noxious agents, tobacco)
- Mechanical trauma (e.g., braces, broken teeth, endotracheal tubeill-fitting dentures, nasogastric tube placement)
- Vomiting

Defining Characteristics
Subjective: verbal reports of dry mouth (xerostomia); oral pain/discomfort.
Objective: atrophy of gums; coated tongue; lack of or decreased salivation; stomatitis; edema of mucosa, halitosis; hemorrhagic gingivitis; hyperemia; oral lesions, plaque, redness, ulcers, vesicles; carious teeth.

Impaired swallowing

Definition: the state in which an individual has decreased ability to voluntarily pass fluids and/or solids from the mouth to the stomach.

Related Factors
- Neuromuscular impairment (decreased or absent gag reflex, decreased strength or excursion of muscles of mastication, perceptual impairment, facial paralysis)
- Mechanical obstruction (edema, tracheostomy tube, tumor)
- Excessive/inadequate salivation
- Fatigue
- Reddened, irritated oropharyngeal cavity
- Limited awareness

Defining Characteristic
Subjective: verbal reports of pain on swallowing.
Objective: observed evidence of difficulty in swallowing (stasis of food in oral cavity, regurgitation of fluids and/or solids through mouth or nose, choking/coughing, pocketing/squirreling of food, food sticking, drooling, standing phlegm, swallowing incoordination, repeated swallows, wet/hoarse voice); evidence of aspiration; dehydration; weight loss.

High risk for aspiration

Definition: the state in which an individual is at risk for entry of gastrointestinal secretions, oropharyngeal secretions, solids, or fluids into tracheobronchial passages.

Related Factors

- Reduced level of consciousness
- Depressed cough and gag reflexes
- Presence of tracheostomy or endotracheal tube
- Incomplete lower esophageal sphincter
- Gastrointestinal tubes
- Tube feedings
- Medication administration
- Situations hindering elevation of upper body
- Increased intragastric pressure
- Increased gastric residual
- Decreased gastrointestinal motility
- Delayed gastric emptying
- Impaired swallowing
- Facial, oral, or neck surgery or trauma
- Wired jaw

Related Nursing Diagnoses

Pain

Ineffective airway clearance

High risk for infection

Self-care deficit

Diversional activity deficit

Impaired home maintenance management

Altered role performance

Social isolation

Impaired social interaction

CASE STUDY

M.W. is a 32-year-old male with complaints of a "sore throat, runny nose and being tired for about 5 days."

Health History

Chief complaint: "sore throat, runny nose and being tired for about 5 days."

Present problem: approximately 5 days ago began complaining of a runny nose and being tired; treated self with Tylenol and over-the-counter antihistamines and decongestants, with no improvement; 2 days ago began complaining of a sore throat, chills, and extreme fatigue; states, "I haven't been able to eat or drink much of anything because my throat hurts so bad;" reported a temperature ranging 100-101 F; also reports a productive cough of a greenish sputum.

Past medical history: reports having several colds each year during the fall and winter seasons; tonsillectomy age 6.

Family history: none contributory.

Social history: denies smoking.

Physical Examination

General: 32-year-old male; ht 5'9", wt 165 lb; BP 110/70, pulse 88, resp 22, temp 101.0° F.

Inspection

Ears: no drainage noted in canals; tympanic membranes pearl gray with landmarks intact.

Nose: mucosa pink, slightly swollen; external surface of nares reddened; small amount thick green discharge noted; nasal pathways occluded, no air exchange noted.

Mouth: oral mucosa and gingivae pink; no lesions.

Throat: pharyngeal walls bright red with yellow-white exudate.

Neck: no redness or swelling noted.

Palpation

Ears: complains of pain during movement of auricles.

Nose: painful to palpation.

Neck: bilateral preauricular, parotid, submandibula and anterior cervical lymph nodes enlarged and painful to palpation; all lymph nodes <1 cm and moveable.

Auscultation: no adventitious breath sounds.

Diagnostic Tests

Throat culture: reveals *Streptococcus pyogenes*.

Problems identified for M.W.

Altered oral mucous membranes related to infection

Defining Characteristics

Subjective: complains of sore throat, difficulty swallowing.

Objective: oral mucosa and gingivae pink; pharyngeal walls bright red with yellow-white exudate; throat culture reveals *Streptococcus pyogenes*.

Impaired swallowing related to reddened irritated oropharynx

Defining Characteristics

Subjective: complains of sore throat, difficulty swallowing; states has not been able to eat or drink because of the sore throat; lymph nodes painful upon palpation.

Objective: oral mucosa and gingivae pink; pharyngeal walls bright red with yellow-white exudate; culture reveals *Streptococcus pyogenes;* bilateral preauricular, parotid, submandibular and anterior cervical lymph nodes enlarged.

Pain related to infectious process of oropharyngeal cavity

Defining Characteristics

Subjective: complains of a sore throat; pain when swallowing; lymph nodes painful upon palpation.

Objective: oral mucosa and gingivae pink; pharyngeal walls bright red with yellow-white exudate; bilateral preauricular, parotid, submandibular, and anterior cervical lymph nodes enlarged.

Sensory/perceptual alteration (olfactory) related to nasal mucosa

Defining Characteristics

Subjective: complains of runny nose; reports nares painful to palpation.

Objective: mucosa pink and slightly swollen; small amount thick green discharge noted; nasal pathways occluded with no air exchange noted.

Other Related Nursing Diagnoses

Sensory/perceptual alteration (gustatory) related to inflammation of oropharyngeal cavity

Ineffective airway clearance related to excess thick secretions

Altered nutrition: less than body requirements related to dysphagia

Hyperthermia related to infectious process

HEALTH PROMOTION

Preservation of hearing

- Avoid placing any objects in the ear
    Clean ears with a washcloth and finger only
    Avoid using bobby pins and cotton-tipped applicators
- Avoid noise levels greater than 85-95 dB
    Promote use of ear protectors in environments with loud noises
    Periodic audiometric screening should be a part of health maintenance policies in industry
    Amplified music should be discouraged and maintained at a reasonable level
- Childhood immunizations should be encouraged, including measles, mumps and rubella (MMR)
- Be aware that many medications have ototoxic effects
- After showering and/or swimming, drain all the water from each ear
    Avoid swimming in contaminated water
    Wear ear plugs if necessary
- Early detection and adequate treatment of ear disorders is recommended
    Seek medical attention promptly when problems arise

Chest and Lungs

NURSING CONSIDERATIONS

Health History

Physiologic needs will always have a higher priority than psychologic or social needs, since they are crucial for survival. Oxygenation is one of the most basic physiologic needs and thus has a very high priority. Patients with respiratory problems will have difficulty focusing on anything else.

Before beginning, quickly assess the patient for signs of acute respiratory distress, such as restlessness, anxiety, inability to follow conversation, or noisy or labored respirations. Intervention may be necessary before any further interview. At this point, the patient's family, friends, or significant other, may be an excellent source of information about the current problem.

When the level of dyspnea and anxiety have decreased, proceed with the full health history. Keep in mind that the patient suffering from hypoxemia, hypoxia, or hypercapnea may have periods of confusion, inattentiveness, or sleepiness. This may alter your patient's ability to answer questions appropriately. Ask questions that can be easily understood and easily answered. You may wish to use direct questions to obtain specific information and avoid any lengthy conversations. It may also be advisable to complete the history in several short interviews to avoid tiring the patient. Set your priorities to determine which components of the health history are necessary and which parts may be deleted at this time.

Physical Examination

To begin your assessment of the respiratory system of the patient, it is important to do an overall assessment of the patient's status. Inspect the skin, paying particular attention to all four extremities for an assessment of peripheral oxygenation. Note any signs of cyanosis that appear as a bluish or purplish color of the skin and mucous membranes caused by a decrease in oxygen levels in the arterial blood.

The location of the cyanosis will determine whether it is central or peripheral cyanosis. Central cyanosis is characterized by a bluish color of the highly vascular areas of the body, such as the buccal mucosa, tongue, lips, and nail beds. This cyanosis is caused by prolonged hypoxia and will effect all body organs.

Peripheral cyanosis is characterized by a bluish tint in the nail beds and occasionally in the lips and does not affect the mucous membranes. These peripheral symptoms can be caused by vascular occlusion and/or vasoconstriction, which can be a result of exposure to cold and hypotension.

Several other indicators of respiratory difficulty should be assessed as well. Finger clubbing and nail thinning can be indicators of respiratory and/or cardiovascular problems. Note any abnormal enlargement of the fingers and toes, and inspect the nails for thinning and ridges. These can be caused by chronic tissue hypoxia.

Nasal flaring provides a larger opening, thereby allowing a greater quantity of air to enter the lungs. Pursed lip breathing provides more force to expel the carbon dioxide during expiration. The use of accessory muscles is an indicator of a need to increase the intake of oxygen and/or removal of carbon dioxide from the lungs. Assess for retractions, which is a sinking of the soft tissues between and around the ribs. This is an indicator of internal intercostal muscle use. The positioning of the patient may also indicate signs of respiratory difficulties. Note whether the patient has a need for several pillows during sleep, assumes a more sitting position and/or three point positioning. These postures allow the diaphragm to drop with less effort and provide for greater expansion of the thoracic cage, thus allowing a greater intake of oxygen with less exertion.

These maneuvers (i.e., nasal flaring, pursed lip breathing, use of accessory muscles and three point positioning), can be seen in a healthy individual after heavy exercise; however, the recovery time for a healthy person will be short.In patients with respiratory disorders such as chronic obstructive pulmonary disease, bronchitis, and cystic fibrosis, these maneuvers can be seen even at rest.

It is vital to provide a warm environment for the patient before beginning the physical assessment. Cold may cause some peripheral cyanosis, and shivering could alter the breathing patterns. A sitting position is preferable in obtaining access to the anterior and posterior thorax. However, for many patient's this position may be difficult. Alternately use the supine semi-Fowlers position to assess the anterior thorax and a lateral or side-lying position for access to the posterior thorax. In any of these positions, the patient should be comfortable. To avoid the constant changing of positions, it may be easier for you and your patient to inspect, palpate, percuss, and auscultate the anterior thorax first and then change positions to assess the posterior aspect.

Basic assessment of respiratory status includes assessment of respiratory motion, that is, rate, type, rhythm, depth, inspiration/expiration ratio, and use of accessory muscles. Note the chest's shape, symmetry, and configuration. So often only inspection and auscultation are used in the clinical setting. It is also important to use palpation and percussion during a basic assessment.

For the patient experiencing respiratory difficulties, it may be difficult to perform, and often prudent to omit, diaphragmatic excursion. To perform this technique the patient must be able to take a deep breath and hold it. If a patient is experiencing moderate to severe respiratory difficulties, this may be difficult and often impossible to do.

Auscultation of breath sounds also becomes difficult in the patient exhibiting respiratory difficulties. It is important to auscultate both the anterior and posterior to obtain a true picture of respiratory status. The lateral breath sounds will be more difficult to obtain and may require some creativity in obtaining them. Optimally, the patient should be in a sitting position with the arms overhead. Having the arms in this position increases the workload of the heart, which can cause an increase in the workload of the respiratory system. It may be easier for you and your patient if you ask the patient to move the arm slightly away from the body, without having to raise it completely overhead.

Performing a health history and physical examination on a patient experiencing respiratory difficultities will produce some degree of fatigue and/or exhaustion for the patient. Your objective is to obtain the necessary information, but the key is to maintain optimal oxygenation during this process. You will need to set your priorities, have patience, and be creative to achieve your goals.

DIAGNOSTIC TESTS

Pulmonary function tests: designed to determine the presence, nature, and extent of pulmonary dysfunction, which can be caused by obstruction, restriction, or a combination of both. The results of pulmonary function studies often reveal abnormalities in the airways, alveoli, and pulmonary vascular bed early in the course of disease when x-ray results and physical examinations are still normal. Also, the location of an airway abnormality may be determined.

Simple spirometer: a basic tool used in routine screening; designed to determine the effectiveness of the various forces involved in the movement of the lungs and chest wall; values obtained will provide quantitative information about the degree of obstruction to air flow and/or restriction of the amount of air that can be inspired; the lung function measurements are compared with the normal values for a person of the same age, sex, and height; race and weight also influence lung function.

Arterial blood gases: requires blood from an artery to assess oxygenation, ventilation, and acid-base balance; arterial blood provides more direct information about ventilatory function; determines the pH, saturation, partial pressure of oxygen, and partial pressure of carbon dioxide.

> **pH**: measures the concentration of hydrogen ions in the blood.
>
> **Partial pressure of oxygen (PaO$_2$)**: reflects the amount of O$_2$ passing from the alveoli into the blood and measures the effectiveness of the lungs to oxygenate the blood.
>
> **Partial pressure of carbon dioxide (PaCO$_2$)**: directly reflects the effectiveness of O$_2$/CO exchange in the lungs.
>
> **Bicarbonate ions (HCO$_3$)**: used to measure the alkalinity or acidity of the blood.
>
> **O$_2$ saturation (SaO$_2$)**: represents a ratio between the actual oxygen content of the hemoglobin compared to the potential maximum O$_2$ carrying capacity of the hemoglobin.
>
> **Fractional concentration of inspired oxygen (FIO2)**: important to keep in mind when interrupting blood gases and/or O$_2$ saturation per pulse oximeter; value is expressed as a percentage, e.g., room air is 21%. This percentage will increase with the administration of O$_2$.

Complete blood cell count (CBC): a basic screening test that provides valuable information about the overall state of health and respiratory status; main elements that relate to the respiratory function are the RBC, Hct, Hgb, WBC, and the differential WBC count.

> **Red blood cells (RBC)**: main function of the RBCs or erythrocytes is to carry oxygen from the lungs to the body tissue and to transfer carbon dioxide from the tissues to the lungs.
>
> **Hemoglobin (Hgb)**: serves as the vehicle for the transportion of oxygen and carbon dioxide.
>
> **Hematocrit (Hct)**: provides information concerning the percentage of RBCs and hydration status.
>
> **White blood cells (WBC)**: function of the WBCs or leukocytes is to fight infection; value provides information concerning the immune response to antigens.
>
> **Neutrophils**: primary function is phagocytosis and reflects the body's reaction to inflammation.
>
> **Eosinophils and basophils**: play a role in the later stages of inflammation and are also active in allergic reactions due to its vasoactive chemicals, histamine and serotonin.
>
> **Monocytes**: the body's second line of defence against infection and reflect phagocytic activity.
>
> **Lymphocytes**: migrate to areas of inflammation in both the early and late stages of inflammation and reflect the activity of antibody production.

Chest X-rays: give valuable information on the condition of the lungs with the property of being able to visualize the lungs, bones, heart, major thoracic vessels, location of invasive lines and presence of fluid, masses, and/or diseases.

Chest tomography: provides information that is not normally provided or confirmed with routine chest x-rays, such as revealing properties of a lung lesion, visualizing certain structures, and revealing small lesions hidden by routine x-rays.

Lung scans: done for 3 reasons: (1) to detect the percentage of the lungs functioning normally, (2) to diagnose and locate pulmonary emboli, and (3) to assess the pulmonary vascular supply by providing information on pulmonary blood flow; 3 types of scans provide information on the perfusion, ventilation, and inhalation ability of the lungs.

Thoracentesis: involves the insertion of a needle into the pleural space for the removal of fluid; removal of fluid is done for diagnostic or therapeutic purposes.

Skin tests: performed to determine immune function and to diagnose pulmonary diseases, distinguishing them from bacterial, fungal, or viral causes; tests include the tuberculin test, Schick test, mumps test, blastomycosis test, and the sweat test.

Bronchoscopy: allows for the visualization of the larynx, trachea, and bronchi; used in the diagnosis and treatment of respiratory disorders.

Pulmonary angiography: pulmonary vascular tree is visualized through use of fluoroscopy and radiopaque dye, allowing for the study of pulmonary circulation.

Respiratory tract cultures: used to diagnose infectious diseases of the respiratory tract; cultures include the sputum, throat, and nose.

NURSING DIAGNOSES

Impaired gas exchange

Definition: the state in which the individual experiences a decrease of oxygen or carbon dioxide between the alveoli of the lungs and the vascular system.

Related Factors
- Altered oxygen supply
- Alveolar-capillary membrane changes
- Altered blood flow
- Altered oxygen-carrying capacity of blood
- Tracheostomy
- Neuromuscular impairment
- Musculoskeletal impairment
- Effects of anesthesia
- Aspiration of foreign matter
- Effects of medication (sedatives, tranquilizers, narcotics)
- Hypoventilation or hyperventilation
- Inhalation of toxic fumes or substances

Defining Characteristics
Subjective: verbal reports of shortness of breath, sense of impending doom.

Objective: irritability, drowsiness, confusion, restlessness, fatigue, lethargy, somnolence, inability to move secretions, hypoxia (PaO$_2$ < 60 mm Hg), hypercapnea (PaCO$_2$ > 45 mm Hg), cyanosis, dyspnea, orthopnea, rales, diminished or absent breath sounds, tachycardia, use of accessory muscles, clubbing of fingers, increased fremitus in lower lobes, dullness percussed over lung fields, decreased or unilateral lung expansion, alteration in respiratory motion (increased rate and depth), three-point positioning, pursed-lip breathing, nasal flaring.

Ineffective airway clearance

Definition: the state in which an individual is unable to clear secretions or obstructions from the respiratory tract to maintain airway patency.

Related Factors

- Decreased energy-fatigue
- Tracheobronchial infection, obstruction, secretions
- Perceptual/cognitive impairment
- Trauma
- Effects of anesthesia
- Effects of infection
- Effects of medications (narcotics, sedatives, tranquilizers, cough suppressants)
- Suppression of cough to avoid pain
- Ineffective cough
- Presence of artificial airway
- Aspiration of foreign matter
- Improper positioning
- Edema in upper airway structures
- Tenacious secretions

Defining Characteristics

Subjective: verbal reports of shortness of breath, fatigue, lack of desire to cough.

Objective: cough (with or without expectoration), dyspnea, rhonchi, crackles, wheezes, alterations in respiratory motion (rate and depth), cyanosis, fever, apnea, fear, anxiety, restlessness, use of accessory muscles, choking, noisy respirations, altered arterial blood gases, labored or irregular breathing, diaphoresis, nasal flaring, stridor.

Ineffective breathing pattern

Definition: the state in which an individual's inhalation or exhalation pattern does not enable adequate pulmonary inflation or emptying.

Related Factors

- Decreased energy
- Decreased lung expansion
- Effects of medications (sedatives, tranquilizers, narcotics)
- Effects of anesthesia
- Effects of obesity
- Immobility, inactivity
- Cognitive impairment
- Musculoskeletal impairment
- Neuromuscular impairment
- Perceptual impairment
- Inflammatory process
- Pain (local, substernal, pleuritic)
- Tracheobronchial obstruction
- Anxiety
- Allergy
- Restrictive dressings

Defining Characteristics

Subjective: verebal reports of shortness of breath, fatigue, pain when breathing, inability to breath, need for oxygen.

Objective: diminished or uneven chest excursion, use of accessory muscles, increased anterioposterior diameter, three-point breathing, pursed-lip breathing, dyspnea, irregular respirations, alteration in respiratory motion (shallow, guarded, rapid), altered arterial blood gases, cough, cyanosis, nasal flaring, prolonged expiratory phase, short inspiratory phase, decreased tidal volume, decreased vital capacity, restlessness, irritability, pleural friction rub, asymmetric chest movements.

Activity intolerance

Definition: the state in which an individual has insufficient physiologic or psychologic energy to endure or complete required or desired activities.

Related Factors

- Generalized weakness
- Sedentary lifestyle
- Imbalance between oxygen supply and demand
- Bedrest or immobility
- Deconditioned status
- Pain
- Electrolyte imbalance
- Hypovolemia
- Malnourishment
- Interrupted sleep
- Impaired sensory or motor function
- Effects of aging
- Effects of medications (sedatives, tranquilizers, narcotics)
- Effects of anesthesia
- Depression
- Lack of motivation
- Cognitive/emotional status changes

Defining Characteristics

Subjective: verbal reports of fatigue or weakness associated with activity, decreased desire or lack of interest in activity, shortness of breath.

Objective: tachycardia with activity, exertional chest pain, dyspnea with activity, exertional discomfort and/or dyspnea, electrocardiographic changes reflecting dysrhythmias or ischemia with activity, alteration in skin color during activity (redness, cyanosis, or pallor), dizziness during activity, worried or uneasy facial expression, impaired ability to change positions or stand or walk without support, weakness, confusion.

Related Nursing Diagnoses

Fluid volume excess
Fatigue
Anxiety
Pain
Sleep pattern disturbance
Altered nutrition: less than body requirements

High risk for infection
Sexual dysfunction
Hyperthermia
Self-care deficit
Altered oral mucous membranes
High risk for aspiration

CASE STUDY

Mr. H. is a 62-year-old male retired railroad worker who sought medical help with complaints of increasing shortness of breath and fatigue within the last 3 to 4 days.

Health History

Chief complaint: increasing shortness of breath and fatigue within last 3 to 4 days.

Present problem: 3 to 4 days before seeking medical attention, began complaining of generalized fatigue and increased dypsnea during activity; unable to climb one flight of stairs without frequent resting; 1 day before seeking help became dypsnec during rest; has three-pillow orthopnea as of 2 days before, along with increasing episodes of paroxysmal nocturnal dyspnea; complains of persistent cough producing large amounts thick tan sputum; states has had a decrease in appetite in the last month.

Past medical history: chronic obstructive pulmonary disease, diagnosed 6 years ago; pneumonia x2, last episode 4 months ago.

Family history: denies history of tuberculosis, emphysema, allergies, or cancer.

Social history: smoked cigarettes, 1 pack/day x35 years; quit 2 years ago; denies use of alcohol.

Physical Examination

General: 62-year-old thin male: ht 6'0", wt 182 lb; BP 140/90, pulse 88, resp 36, temp 100.2° F.

Inspection: in sitting position leaning forward on bedside table (3-point positioning); resp 36, regular and labored; prolonged active expiration; anteroposterior diameter = transverse diameter (barrel chest); supraclavicular and intercostal retractions noted with intercostal bulging with expiration; using accessory muscles during respirations; tactile fremitus equal bilaterally, increasing in lower lobes; chest expansion symmetrical, costal angle greater that 90 degrees; nail base angle greater than 160 degrees (nail clubbing); nasal flaring and pursed lip breathing noted; lips and nail beds slightly cyanotic.

Palpation: no masses, tenderness, or crepitus.

Percussion: dullness noted bilateral lower lobes with hyperresonance in all remaining lobes; diaphragmatic excursion deferred.

Auscultation: breath sounds diminished all lobes; course crackles noted in bilateral lower lobes.

Diagnostic Tests

Chest x-ray: shows infiltration in bilateral lower lobes. All other lobes clear.

Complete blood cell count (CBC): Hgb 12.1 g/dl; Hct 39.0%;
RBC 5.2 10/mm; WBC 15,000/mm; neutrophils 53%; lymphocytes 48%; monocytes 10%, basophils 2%, eosinophils 3%

Arterial blood gases (ABG): pH 7.32; PaO_2 72 mmHg; $PaCO_2$ 49 mmHg; HCO3 21 mEq/L; SaO_2 83%; FIO2 room air

Lung function studies: decreased lung volumes; increased resistance; decreased compliance.

Problems identified for Mr. H.

Ineffective airway clearance related to large amounts of tenacious secretions

Defining Characterisitcs

Subjective: complains of dyspnea, fatigue and a productive cough.

Objective: productive cough producing large amounts of thick, tan secretions; infiltrations in bilateral lower lobes on chest x-ray; crackles bilateral lower lobes; febrile; dyspnea, tachypnea; use of accessory muscles; altered arterial blood gases.

Impaired gas exchange related to alveolar-capillary membrane changes secondary to the inflammatory process

Defining Characteristics

Subjective: complains of dyspnea, fatigue with exertion and rest and paroxysmal nocturnal dyspnea.

Objective: history of chronic obstructive pulmonary disease; history of pneumonia, history of smoking; cyanosis; 3-pillow orthopnea; diminished breath sounds; crackles bilaterial lower lobes; increased fremitus in lower lobes; use of accessory muscles; clubbing of fingers; dullness percussed over lower lobes, barrel chest; 3-point positioning, nasal flaring, pursed-lip breathing; decreased lung volumes; altered ABGs, (hypoxia, hypercapnea); infiltrations on chest x-ray; altered Hgb and Hct.

Ineffective breathing pattern related inflammatory process

Defining Characteristics

Subjective: complains of dyspnea and fatigue.

Objective: dyspnea; productive cough; tachypnea; increased anteroposterior diameter; use of accessory muscles; nasal flaring; pursed-lip breathing; 3 point positioning; alteration in respiratory motion; prolonged expiratory phase; decreased lung volumes; increased airway resistance; decreased compliance.

Other nursing diagnoses to consider

Hyperthermia related to inflammatory process

Altered nutrition: less than body requirements related to anorexia and dyspnea

Activity intolerance related to imbalance between oxygen supply and demand

Fatigue related to increased metabolic demands secondary to inflammatory process and decreased respiratory reserve

HEALTH PROMOTION

Risk factors associated with respiratory disability

- Gender: greater risk for men
- Age: risk increases with age
- Race: chronic obstructive pulmonary disease is slightly more frequent in whites
- Heredity: family history of asthma, cystic fibrosis, tuberculosis and other contagious disease
- Smoking
- Inactivity: voluntary or involuntary
- Occupation: exposure to asbestos, dust, or other pulmonary irritants and toxic inhalants
- Obesity
- Difficulty swallowing for any reason
- Weakened chest muscles for any reason
- History of frequent respiratory infections

Preventing respiratory infections

- Maintain a proper diet (nutritious, well-balanced)
- Drink at least 6 to 8 glasses of water each day
- Take a vitamin supplement each day
- Obtain plenty of sleep (6-8 hours per night)
- Stay away from persons who have a cold or flu, if possible

- Wash your hands frequently, especially: after handling soiled tissues, after using the bathroom, before putting anything in your mouth, and after handling anything out in public
- Avoid air pollution (tobacco smoke, wood or oil smoke, car exhaust and industrial pollution)
- Avoid smoking
- Rinse your oral inhaler after each use
- Take your medicine exactly as prescribed
- Consult your physician about flu vaccines

Heart and Blood Vessels

NURSING CONSIDERATIONS

Health History

Cardiovascular disease is the most common cause of death and most prevalent health care problem in the United States today. Because of these facts, the cardiovascular assessment becomes a very important one. It is essential that the health care provider be proficient in assessing the cardiac health of the patient.

As with the respiratory system, any involvement of the cardiovascular system produces varying degrees of anxiety in the patient. The mere mention of any type of cardiac abnormality sends a wave of fear and panic through most of us. This is important to remember as you obtain your health history and physical examination. Use discretion, be calm, explain everything, and be supportive.

Your first priority is to establish the presence of any signs/symptoms that may place the patient in immediate danger, such as chest pain, dyspnea, severe tachycardia, extreme hypotension or hypertension. If any of these conditions are present, they will require immediate attention before completing the health history.

For a patient who has or has had chest pain, the textbook does an excellent job of including all the information that is necessary to obtain from that patient. It is, however, important to allow the patients to verbalize their symptoms in their own words. Discomfort/pain can be described in many different ways, from a dull ache to crushing or stabbing pain. A description of the location of the discomfort is also important. The classic textbook sign of a myocardial infarction in males is chest pain that may or may not radiate to the left arm. However, there are many documented cases of an infarction with discomfort verbalized in a variety of areas, such as jaw, teeth, elbow, upper back, stomach, right arm. Only after the patient has described the discomfort in his own words is it advisable to prompt him or her to obtain more information. A few examples of this:

Can you describe this feeling?
Did it move anywhere?
Was this feeling anywhere else?
Would you describe this feeling as discomfort or more likea pain?
Did you feel dizzy at the any time?
What were you doing when this feeling started?

With cardiovascular disease a great deal of time and resources are devoted to the promotion and education for a healthy heart. During the health history, the health care provider needs to assess the patient's personal habits and knowledge in this area. This then provides a basis for further education and lifestyle changes. These topics should include sleep patterns, use of tobacco and/or alcohol, nutrition, exercise, and stress.

Physical Examination

A cardiovascular assessment should be organized. Begin with an overall evaluation of the patient, assessing general appearance, vital signs and related body structures. Assessing general appearance consists of height, weight and muscle composition. The patient should appear well developed, well nourished, alert, and energetic. Note any signs of cardiac cachexia, such as weakness and muscle wasting in the upper arms, thighs, and chest wall.

Evaluation of vital signs included: temperature, pulse rate, respiration rate, blood pressure and pulse pressure. An elevated body temperature increases metabolism, which increases the cardiac work load. A possible cause may be a cardiovascular inflammation or infection. Assess the pulse rate for rate and regularity. Evaluate respiratory status: rate, rhythm, type, depth, and use of accessory muscles. Many respiratory conditions accompany cardiovascular disorders. Assess the patient's blood pressure. An elevated blood pressure may result from hypertension or emotional stress associated with external factors. Allow the patient to relax for approximately 5 to10 minutes following an elevated reading, and then repeat the blood pressure. After obtaining the blood pressure, calculate the pulse pressure (the difference between the systolic pressure and the diastolic pressure). The pulse pressure reflects arterial pressure during the resting phase of the cardiac cycle.

A patient with a cardiovascular disorder may exhibit signs of illness in other parts of the body, since the cardiovascular system affects many other body systems. These areas included skin, hair, nails, and eyes.

The skin should be evaluated for color, turgor, temperature, and moisture. Inspect for the presence of cyanosis. Assess the skin of the extremities and the nail beds for signs of peripheral cyanosis and the underside of the tongue, buccal mucosa, and conjunctiva for signs of central cyanosis. Evaluate the skin turgor (resiliency), which reflects the elasticity and water content of the skin and subcutaneous tissues. The skin should be warm and dry. Cool, clammy skin results from vasoconstriction, which occurs when the cardiac output is low, such as in the case of shock. Warm, moist skin results from vasodilation, which occurs when the cardiac output is high, as with exercise. While inspecting the skin, note the presence of hair and the distribution. Lack of normal body hair on the arms and/or legs may indicate diminished arterial blood flow to these areas.

Nails should be assessed for color, shape, thickness, and symmetry. Fingernails normally appear smooth, rounded, and pinkish and have no markings. Peripheral vascular disease can produce nail depressions, pitting, longitudinal striations, thinning, and brittleness. A bluish color in the nail beds indicates peripheral cyanosis. Assess capillary refill in the fingernails to estimate the rate of peripheral blood flow. Note the nail base angle for signs of clubbing, which indicates chronic tissue hypoxia.

Assessment of the eyes may provide clues to cardiovascular difficulties. The eyes should be clear and bright. Inspect the eyelids for xanthelasmas, which are raised, yellowish plaques resulting from lipid deposits, and can indicate hyperlipidemia, a risk factor of cardiac disease. Note the color of the sclera. A yellowish color may indicate jaundice which usually is a result of liver congestion and may be caused by right-sided heart failure. Inspect the eyes for arcus senilis. For patient's over 60, it is a common effect of aging; however, if present before age 40, it may indicate a lipid disorder. Using the opthalmoscope, examine the retina for structural changes, such as narrowing or blocking of a vein, and hemorrhages, which may indicate hypertension.

The use of a proper sequence during any examination is advised. The usual sequence begins with inspection, palpation, percussion, and finally auscultation. However, it is necessary to remember that it is not the sequence that has the priority, but the patient's comfort. To conserve time and patient energy, you may wish to combine or reorder the techniques.

One aspect of a physical examination that is often neglected is the adjustment of room temperature before beginning. Since your patient's chest will be exposed, the room should be warm. This will not only be more comfortable, but also prevent shivering, which can interfere with the auscultation of the heart sounds. Also, if the room is cold enough, vasoconstriction will occur and alter the results of capillary refill, skin temperature, peripheral pulse quality, heart rate, and blood pressure.

With this examination, it is necessary to expose the chest, which may cause embarrassment to the female patient. Discuss the examination process beforehand, and provide drapes throughout the examination. If your patient has large breasts, it may become necessary for you or the patient to move the left breast if it interferes with palpation and auscultation of the heart. Explanations, sensitivity, and discretion are required in these circumstances.

Percussion of the heart is more frequently being omitted from the examination process. Its purpose is to locate the borders of the heart providing information about the heart size, which is better achieved by chest x-rays. The presence of breast tissue often complicates percussion and only serves to create further embarrassment.

After completing the health history and physical examination, the health care provider is in an excellent position to plan and implement the necessary education and lifestyle changes necessary to restore the patient to maximum cardiovascular health. Many hospital programs and public associations were created to assist the health care provider and patient with this goal.

DIAGNOSTIC TESTS

Electrolytes

Potassium: the major electrolyte (cation) of intracellular fluid and the primary buffer within the cell itself; plays an important role in nerve conduction muscle function, and maintains acid base balance and osmotic pressure; along with calcium and magnesium, potassium controls the rate and force of contraction of the heart, thereby effecting the cardiac output (Hyper or hypokalemia can be noted on an electrocardiogram.).

Calcium: used by the body in processes such as muscular contraction, cardiac function, transmission of nerve impulses, and blood clotting.

Magnesium: necessary for the use of adenosine triphosphate (ADP) as a source of energy; essential for carbohydrate metabolism, protein synthesis, nucleic acid synthesis and the contraction of muscular tissue; magnesium and calcium are closely tied together, therefore a deficiency in either one has significant effect on the metabolism of the other.

Creatinine phosphokinase (CPK) and isoenzymes: an enzyme found in high concentrations in the heart muscle, skeletal muscle and smaller concentrations in the brain; serum CPK levels rise with injury to these cells; test is used to detect injury predominantly to the myocardium and muscle. CPK can be divided into 3 isoenzymes, *MM*, *BB*, and *MB*, which can be used to determine more specifically where the damage has occured.

- elevation in CPK-MM is an indication of skeletal muscle damage.
- The CPK-MB level that is contained in cardiac muscle, provides more definitive information of myocardial cell damage death, specifically the degree of myocardial infarction and the onset of the infarction.
- CPK-BB are found predominantly in the brain tissue, gastrointestinal and genitourinary tracts, and lung tissue.

Lactic acid dehydrogenase (LDH): an enzyme found in several body tissues, especially the heart, liver, kidneys, skeletal muscle, brain and lungs; useful in confirming a myocardial or pulmonary infarct; Since the LDH level by itself is nonspecific, it is necessary to consider this value in conjunction with other test findings.

Cholesterol: a lipid required for the production of steroids, bile acids and cellular membranes; high levels of cholesterol are associated with atherosclerosis and increased risk of coronary artery disease; used to evaluate the potential of such a risk.

Electrocardiogram (ECG, EKG): a recording of the electrical impulses that stimulate the heart to contract; each normal heartbeat begins with an electrical impulse that originates in a specialized area of the right atrium producing a weak electrical current that spreads through the heart causing a contraction; waveform on a ECG represents this single electrical impulse as it travels through the heart; recording is used to identify abnormal heart rhythms (dysrhythmias), the sizes of the cardiac chambers, and to diagnose certain abnormalities.

Ambulatory Electrocardiography (Holter Monitor): portable device that records the electrical activity of the heart as the patient continues normal daily activities; is useful for patient's with suspected rhythm disturbance, monitoring pacemaker function and monitoring the effects of antiarrhythmic therapy.

Stress/exercise testing: provides information about the patient's heart function in response to physical stress. Information on the myocardial response to increased oxygen demands and the adequacy of coronary blood flow is provided; used to evaluate the possible occurance of chest pain in a patient suspected of having coronary artery disease, determine the limits of safe exercise, detect labial or exercise-related hypertension, detect intermittent claudication and/or to evaluate the effectiveness of antianginal or antiarrhythmic therapy.

Echocardiogram: noninvasive examination used to evaluate the internal structures of the heart and great vessels; position, size, movements of the valves and chambers, and velocity of blood flow can be determined by means of reflected ultrasound.

Cardiac catheterization and Angiography: an invasive procedure used to study and diagnose defects of the heart; by inserting arterial and venous catheters carrying contrast material into the right and left sides of the heart, the chambers, valves, great vessels, and coronary arteries can be visualized; in addition, pressure measurements and blood volumes can be obtained to evaluate cardiac function and provide information concerning valve patency; blood samples can also be obtained directly from the heart to measure oxygen content and saturation.

Chest X-rays: provides information about the heart, lungs, and great vessels such as anatomic position and gross structures; silhouette seen on x-ray gives an indication of size of the major cardiac structures.

NURSING DIAGNOSES

Decreased cardiac output

Definition: the state in which the blood pumped by an individual's heart is sufficiently reduced to the extent it is inadequate to meet the needs of the body's tissues. This state places an individual at risk for experiencing cardiovascular, cerebral, or respiratory symptoms, resulting from an insufficient volume of blood being pumped by the heart.

Related Factors
- Reduction in stroke volume as a result of (one or more of the following):

Electrical Factors/Defects
- Alteration in rate
- Alteration in rhythm
- Alteration in conduction
- Pacemaker failure

Mechanical Factors/Defects
- Alteration in preload
- Decreased venous return
- Alteration in myocardial contractility
- Alteration in afterload
- Alteration in systemic vascular resistance
- Alteration in inotropic changes within the heart

Structural Factors/Defects
- Secondary to congenital abnormalities
- Trauma
- Ventricular-septal rupture
- Ventricular aneurysm
- Papillary muscle rupture
- Valvular disease
- Valvular dysfunction
- Decreased ventricular filling

Defining Characteristics

Subjective: verbal reports of fatigue, syncope, anorexia, vertigo, weakness, angina, palpitations, dyspnea, "skipped beats", activity intolerance.

Objective: variations in hemodynamic readings, dysrhythmias; electrocardiographic changes, fatigue, jugular vein distention; cyanosis or pallor of skin and/or mucous membranes, cold and/or clammy skin; mental status changes; cough; frothy sputum; dyspnea; orthopnea; altered blood gases; crackles; abnormal heart sounds; decreased peripheral pulses; syncope; tachycardia; oliguria; anuria; restlessness; edema of trunk/sacrum/extremities; sudden weight gain.

Pain

Definition: the state in which an individual experiences and reports the presence of severe discomfort or an uncomfortable sensation.

Related Factors

- Inflammatory process
- Imbalance of myocardial oxygen supply and demand
- Trauma
- Peripheral ischemia
- Surgical incision

Defining Characteristics

Subjective: verbal report of pain, discomfort, uncomfortable sensation, nausea

Objective: guarding, holding chest, facial mask or grimacing, increased heart rate, increased respiration, increased blood pressure, pallor, anxiety, restlessness, nausea, vomiting, diaphoresis, moaning, crying, pacing, self focusing, narrowed focus, panic, impaired thought processes

Altered tissue perfusion (cardiopulmonary, peripheral)

Definition: the state in which an individual experiences a decrease in nutrition or oxygenation at the cellular level due to a deficit in capillary blood supply

Related Factors

- Interruption of arterial flow
- Interruption of venous flow
- Hypervolemia
- Hypovolemia
- Trauma
- Prolonged sitting/standing
- Immobolization
- Oxygen/carbon dioxide exchange problems
- Decreased cardiac output
- Increased peripheral vascular resistance

Defining Characteristics

Subjective:

Cardiopulmonary: verbal reports of chest pain, palpitations, dyspnea

Peripheral: verbal reports of edema in extremities, cold feet, numbness/tingling in feet.

Objective:

Cardiopulmonary: chest pain, tachycardia, increased respirations, dyspnea, altered pulse pressure

Peripheral:

- Arterial
- Decreased/diminished pulses
- Decreased capillary refill
- Muscle wasting
- Bruits present
- Shiny/taut skin
- Claudication
- Cool/cold extremities
- Pallor/cyanosis/mottled/rubor in color
- Diminished/absence of hair
- Blood pressure changes in extremities
- Ulcerated skin/poorly healing areas
- Slow growing, dry, thick, brittle nails
- Altered sensory or motor function
- Numbness/tingling/burning
- Tissue necrosis/gangrene
- Venous
- Warm, flushed extremities
- Aching, tightness
- Edema
- Engorged veins
- Brown discoloration
- Positive Homan's sign

Activity Intolerance

Definition: the state in which an individual has insufficient physiologic energy to endure or complete required or desired activities.

Related Factors
- Sedentary life style
- Bed rest/inactivity
- Decreased cardiac output
- Myocardial ischemia
- Hypoxemia
- Deconditioned status
- Electrolyte imbalance
- Hypovolemia
- Imbalance between oxygen supply and demand
- Presence of circulatory problems
- Diminished/decreased cardiac reserve

Defining Characteristics

Subjective: Verbal reports of chest pain with exertion, dyspnea, fatigue, generalized weakness, dyspnea on exertion, decreased ability to perform daily activities

Objective: exertional tachycardia, dyspnea, fatigue/weakness with activity, electrocardiographic changes reflecting dysrhythmias or ischema with activity

---

Related Nursing Diagnoses
Anxiety
Altered health maintainence
Knowledge deficit
Ineffective individual coping
Noncompliance
Fluid volume excess
Impaired gas exchange
Altered nutrition: less than body requirements
Self-care deficit

CASE STUDY

Mr. W. is a 57-year-old male, attorney, who sought medical attention with complaints of persisting chest discomfort

Health History

Chief complaint: persisting chest discomfort unrelieved by rest.

Present problem: approximately 3 months prior to seeking attention, began noting vague chest pains during activity, usually relieved with rest; 2 days before began experiencing chest discomfort radiating to left arm, neck, and jaw area; discomfort subsides after 20 to 30 minutes of rest; accompanying the discomfort is slight dyspnea, palpitations, and diaphoresis; denies any nausea, vomiting, lightheadedness or dizziness.

Past medical history: no previous cardiac history; appendectomy 14 years ago.

Family history: father died from heart disease, age 67; mother alive and well; brother diagnosed with hypertension, age 42.

Social history: smokes cigarettes, 1 pack/day x 20 years; drinks approximately 3 beers over the weekend; trying to maintain a low fat diet but eats 2 meals/day out; works long hours; states he is under alot of stress at home and work; plays racquetball 3x/week

Physical Examination

General: 57-year-old male: ht 5'11", wt 225 lb, BP right 160/98, left 152/98, pulse 96 (irregular), resp 32, temp 99.2°F

Inspection: supine with head of bed elevated 45 degrees; anxious; skin pink, no cyanosis, slightly diaphoretic; capillary refill <2 seconds; no clubbing; slight dyspnea at rest noted; no jugular venous pulsations noted; no heaves/lifts or thoracic deformities.

Palpation: apical impulse palpated at 5th intercostal space, 2 cm left midclavicular line; no heaves/thrills; all peripheral pulses 2+, irregular; no edema noted.

Percussion: deferred

Auscultation: S1, S2, without splitting; S3 noted at apex, early diastole, low pitch; no murmurs; lungs clear all lobes

Diagnostic Tests

ECG: changes noted consistent with myocardial injury (ST elevations and Q wave formation)

CPK: 82 U/ml (elevated)

CPK-MB: 32% (elevated)

LDK: 104 U/L (elevated)

Potassium: 3.7 mEq/L

Calcium: 9.2 mg/dl

Magnesium: 1.5 mEq/L

Cholesterol: 320 mg/dl (elevated)

Chest x-ray: normal, no signs of cardiomegaly

Echocardiogram: abnormal right ventricular wall motion

Problems identified for Mr. W.

Pain related to imbalance of myocardial oxygen supply and demand

Defining Characteristics

Subjective: complaints of persisting chest discomfort

Objective: anxiety; diaphoretic, increased blood pressure, increased heart rate

Decreased cardiac output related to reduction in stroke volume as a result of electrical, mechanical and structural defects.

Defining Characteristics

Subjective: complains of chest pain; dyspnea; palpitations

Objective: slight dyspnea; presence of S3; tachycardia, anxiety, electrocardiographic changes; increased levels CPK, CPK-MB, LDH

Altered tissue perfusion (cardiopulmonary) related to interruption of arterial flow

Defining Characteristics

Subjective: complains of chest pain; palpitations

Objective: chest pain; tachycardia; increased respiratory rate; dyspnea

Other nursing diagnoses to consider

Activity intolerance related to imbalance between oxygen supply and demand

Potential fluid volume excess related to . . .

Potential impaired gas exchange related to . . .

HEALTH PROMOTION

Risk factors associated with cardiac disease

- Heredity: family history of cardiovascular disease, diabetes, hyperlipidemia, hypertension.
- Gender: men more than women, and at a younger age; women before menopause have a one in six chance as men in the same age group; after menopause, the difference narrows until approximately age 75 when women become as likely as men to develop cardiac disease.
- Race: Black men under the age of 55 and Black women of all ages have increased incidence of hypertension than do caucasians, which increases the risk of cardiac disease in Blacks.
- Age: the death rate from cardiac disease increases with age.
- Hypertension: treated or untreated (it is more prevalent in Black, elderly, obese persons and in those taking oral contraceptives).
- Diabetes mellitus
- Smoking
- Hyperlipidemia
- Obesity
- Inactivity
- Stress: personalities that typically exhibit chronic overreaction to stress; an exaggerated sense of urgency; excessive aggressiveness, competitiveness, and hostility; and compulsive striving for achievement.
- Diet: a diet high in cholesterol and staurated fats may lead to hyperlipidemia and hypertension; high caffeine intake may contribute to hypertension and dysrhythmias.
- Oral contraceptives: risk of hypertension is greater in women using oral contraceptives
- Alcohol: heavy drinking can cause hypertension that can lead to heart failure.

Breasts and Axillae

NURSING CONSIDERATIONS

Health History

The American Cancer Society estimates that one out of every 9 women in the United States will develop breast cancer at some time in her life; only 1% of all breast cancers occur in men. Every woman should consider herself at risk for this type of cancer. The good news is that due to new and better treatment, combined with early detection, many women who develop cancer will go on to live full lives. Every woman should know the signs of breast cancer and know how to detect it early.

There are several tools that should be used for the early detection of cancer. These include monthly breast self-examinations, examination by a trained health professional, and mammography. During the health history, it is important to obtain information such as (1) does the woman/man perform breast self-examination, (2) is it done consistently and at the same time each month, and (3) when was the last mammogram and are they done on a regular basis.

The physical examination offers a great opportunity to not only perform a thorough breast examination, but also to assess the patient's technique. If through the health history you have determined a lack of knowledge concerning the examination, this is an excellent time to begin your teaching.

Since this cancer is so prevalent, it is vital that we as professionals make every attempt to provide the necessary information and teaching to all of our patients.

The nurse should prepare the patient for the health history by explaining the purpose of the interview. This explanation should state that some of the questions may seem very personal, but the information is necessary. Discussing the breast may be embarrassing for some patients, so ensure a comfortable interview environment that offers privacy and freedom from interruptions. Perform the interview before the physical examination while the patient is still fully clothed.

Remember that female breasts are significantly associated with sexuality so that any threat to the breast can threaten a woman's body image and feelings of personal worth. This directly affects relationships with others.

Physical Examination

Before beginning your examination, ensure privacy, provide explanations, a comfortable room temperature, and present with a gentle and objective approach. Be attentive to your patient's comfort, allow sufficient time for a thorough assessment and proceed systematically. The textbook does an excellent job exploring the psychologic aspects of a breast examination.

DIAGNOSTIC TESTS

Breast self-examination: done by the women herself encompassing a series of steps that are done to detect breast cancer as early as possible. This examination needs to be done each month, at the same time each month.

Professional breast examination: same examination as a self-examination but done by a professional; is recommended that this be done on a yearly basis.

Mammography: a low-dose breast x-ray used to find cancers too small to be felt; can also reveal other breast changes that may signal a very early breast cancer; women over 40 years of age need to have regular mammograms whether they have symptoms or not.

NURSING DIAGNOSES

Body Image Disturbance

Definition: the state in which an individual experiences a negative or distorted perception of the body.

Related Factors
- Physical trauma/mutilation
- Pregnancy
- Physical change caused by biochemical agents (drugs)
- Dependence on machine
- Effects of loss of body part(s)
- Effects of loss of body function with regard to age, sex, developmental level or basic human needs
- Psychosocial difficulties
- Cultural or spiritual difficulties
- Maturational changes

Defining Characteristics
Subjective: verbal reports of change in lifestyle; fear of rejection or reaction by others; preoccupation with change or loss; feelings of helplessness, hopelessness, or powerlessness; refusal to verify actual change; refusal to participate in self-care; negative feelings about self; focuses on past strength, function, or appearance; guilt or shame.

Objective: missing body part; actual change in structure and/or function; hiding or overexposing body part; trauma to nonfunctioning part; change in ability to estimate spatial relationship of body to environment; extension of body boundary to incorporate environmental objects; preoccupation with change or loss; change in social involvement; not looking at or touching body part.

Ineffective individual coping

Definition: the state in which an individual demonstrates impaired adaptive behaviors and problem-solving abilities.

Related Factors

- Situational crises
- Maturational crises
- Personal vulnerability
- Inadequate coping skills
- Unrealistic perceptions
- Multiple stressors/life changes
- Major changes in lifestyle
- Inadequate relaxation/leisure activities
- Low self-esteem
- Unmet expectations
- Poor nutrition
- Work overload
- Too many deadlines
- Unrealistic perceptions
- Inadequate support systems
- Little or no exercise
- Knowledge deficit regarding therapeutic regimen, disease process, and/or prognosis
- Sensory overload
- Severe pain
- Overwhelming threat to self
- Impairment to nervous system

Defining Characteristics

Subjective: verbal reports of inability to cope; inability to meet expectations; inability to ask for help; inability to problem solve; verbal manipulation, reports of chronic worry/anxiety/depression; lack of appetite; chronic fatigue; insomnia; general irritability.

Objective: insomnia; physical inactivity; substance abuse; alteration in societal participation, destructive behavior toward self or others; inappropriate use of defense mechanisms; change in usual communication patterns; inability to meet or take responsibility for basic needs; exaggerated fear of pain, death; general irritability; high rate of injuries or illnesses; frequent headaches/neckaches; indecisiveness, overeating; excessive smoking; excessive drinking; irritable bowel; poor self-esteem; lack of assertive behaviors.

Anxiety

Definition: vague uneasy feeling whose source is often nonspecific or unknown to the individual.

Related Factors

- Threat to self-concept
- Situational and/or maturational crisis
- Interpersonal transmission and contagion
- Threat of death (perceived or actual)
- Threat to or change in health status
- Threat to or change in role functioning
- Threat to or change in environment
- Threat to or change in interaction patterns
- Threat to or change in socioeconomic status
- Unmet needs
- Unconscious conflict about essential values and goals of life

Defining Characteristics

Subjective: verbal reports of increased tension; apprehension; uncertainty; feeling of being scared; feeling of inadequacy; shakiness; fear of unspecific consequences; overexcitedness; increased helplessness; regret; feeling of being rattled; distress; jitteriness.

Objective: sympathetic stimulation-cardiovascular excitation, superficial vasoconstriction, pupil dilation; restlessness; insomnia; glancing about; poor eye contact; trembling; hand tremors; extraneous movements-footshuffling, hand and/or arm movements; facial tension; voice quivering; focus on self; increased wariness; increased perspiration.

Fear

Definition: the state in which the individual experiences feelings of dread related to an identifiable source perceived as dangerous.

Related Factors

- Sensory impairment, deprivation, or overload
- Pain
- Effects of loss of body part or function
- Effects of chronic disabling illness
- Language barrier
- Threat of death, actual or perceived
- Anticipation of events posing a threat to self-esteem
- Phobias
- Feelings of failure
- Knowledge deficit
- Learned response, conditioning
- Loss of significant other
- Separation from support system

Defining Characteristics

Subjective: verbal reports of increased tension, apprehension, impulsiveness, decreased self-assurance, afraid, scared, terrified, panic, jittery, nausea, "heart beating fast", feelings of loss of control.
Objective: increased alertness, concentration on source, wide-eyed, aggressive behavior, withdrawn, sympathetic stimulation (increased heart rate, flushing, pupil dilation, vomiting, diarrhea, diaphoresis), voice tremors, urinary frequency, insomnia, increased questioning/verbalization.

Self-esteem disturbance

Definition: the state in which an individual has negative self-evaluation/feelings about self or self capabilities, which may be directly or indirectly expressed.

Related Factors

- Effects of loss of body part(s)
- Effects of loss of body function
- "Failure" at life events (e.g., loss of job, divorce)
- Effects of aging

Defining Characteristics

Subjective: verbal reports of self-negating; expressions of shame/guilt; evaluates self as unable to deal with events; rationalizes away/rejects positive feedback and exaggerates negative feedback about self.
Objective: hesitant to try new things/situations; denial of problems obvious to others; projection of blame/responsibility for problems; rationalizes personal failures; hypersensitive to criticism; grandiosity; lack of follow-through; nonparticipation in therapy; self-destructive behavior, lack of eye contact.

Related Nursing Diagnoses

Ineffective breastfeeding
Altered family processes
Anticipatory grieving
Dysfunctional grieving
Altered health maintenance
Hopelessness

Knowledge deficit
Personal identity disturbance
Powerlessness
Impaired social interaction
Social isolation
Spiritual distress

CASE STUDY

D.B is a 62-year-old black female who came to the hospital with a diagnosis of left breast mass.

Health History

Chief complaint: "The doctor found a mass in my left breast."

Present problem: 3 days before admission during a yearly company physical examination, the doctor noted a lump in her left breast; was told she needed an immediate breast biopsy with the possibility of a mastectomy.

Past medical history: no previous breast history; hypertension managed by diuretics and diet; has had two uncomplicated deliveries; one spontaneous abortion, age 32; menopause completed at age 53 without problems.

Family history: Mother died age 56 of breast cancer; father alive and well; no siblings.

Social history: Verbalized that she is aware of breast self-examination but has never performed it. "I feel so bad. If only I had been doing it. I should have found this myself." States husband is supportive but she is afraid to tell him. "What will he think of me when he hears I may have to have my breast removed? I am not sure I will be able to look in the mirror if they remove my breast. I don't know what to think or do."

Physical Examination

General: 62 year-old-female: tt 5'4", wt 163 lb; BP 102/72, pulse 86, resp 22, temp 98.0° F.

Inspection: breasts symmetric when sitting and with arms down; bilateral nipples flat; no lesions or discharge noted; with arms elevated, right breast elevates, left breast remains fixed; dimple noted in left breast, 2:00 position; leaning forward reveals right breast falls free while left breast flattens.

Palpation: right breast feels soft and granular throughout with no mass; left breast soft and granular, with large, stony hard mass approximately 3mm in diameter in outer quadrant; lump noted 2:00 position, 3 cm from nipple; borders irregular; mass fixed to tissues; denies pain with palpation; no palpable nodes on the right; one firm, palpable lymph node in center of left axilla.

Diagnostic Tests

Mammography: shows a mass, left breast; 5 x 4 x 2 cm, at 2:00 position, 3 cm from nipple; right breast no masses seen.

Problems identified for D.B.

Body image disturbance related to the potential loss of a body part

Defining Characteristics

Subjective: verbalized fear of rejection by her husband; preoccupation with the loss of her breast; verbalized negative feelings about self if her breast is removed; feelings of guilt for not performing breast self-examination and not finding the mass herself.

Objective: presence of a large mass in the left breast and the potential for a mastectomy.

Ineffective individual coping related to situational crisis (potential loss of her left breast)

Defining Characteristics

Subjective: verbalizes anxiety concerning present situation; inability to problem solve.

Objective: presence of large mass in the left breast and the potential for a mastectomy.

Self-esteem disturbance related to cognitive perceptual factors

Defining Characteristics

Subjective: evaluation of self as unable to deal with events; verbalization of negative feelings about self; expressions of guilt; difficulty making decisions.

Objective: presence of large mass in the left breast and the potential for a mastectomy.

Fear related to anticipation of evens posing a threat to self and self-esteem

Defining Characteristics

Subjective: states she is afraid to tell her husband; states she may not be able to look in the mirror is the breast is removed

Other problems to consider for D.B.:

Knowledge deficit: breast self-examination

Anxiety

Altered health maintenance

Altered sexuality patterns

Impaired social interaction

HEALTH PROMOTION

Risk factors associated with breast cancer

- Age
- Early menarche (before age 12)
- Late menopause (after age 50)
- Nulliparity
- Late age at birth of first child (after age 30)
- Personal history of premalignant mastopathy
- Personal history of ovarian, endometrial, or colon cancer
- Family history of breast cancer
- Diet high in animal fats
- Obesity
- Smoking

Preventing breast cancer

- Monthly breast self-examination
- Yearly examination by a trained professional
- Screening (baseline) mammogram between ages 35-30
- Screening (baseline) mammogram at age 30 if a family history of breast cancer is present

Signs of Breast Cancer

- Lump or thickening in the breast or arm-pit
- Change in the breast skin color, dimpling or puckering
- Nipple discharge
- Change in the size or shape of the breast
- Change in the direction the nipple points

Abdomen

NURSING CONSIDERATIONS

Health History

Even though the patient has no overt gastrointestinal (GI) problem, questions should cover dietary intake, appetite, digestion, bowel elimination patterns, medication use, urinary elimination patterns, and history of past and present GI problems. All complaints need to be fully explored, even the ones the patient may dismiss as unimportant, such as "heartburn," "upset stomach," and "too much gas." Such complaints could indicate a serious underlying problem.

The kidney has a profound effect on all systems in the body and on the patient's overall health. Because of the interactions between the urinary system and other body systems, a disorder originating in the urinary system may disrupt the function in other systems and vice versa. It is for these reasons that the nurse must always assess for signs and symptoms of urinary disorders, even if the patient does not have any complaints in this area. Such signs and symptoms may include hematuria, cloudy urine, incontinence, frequency, hesitancy, abdominal pain, edema, and urgency. These indicate a need for further in-depth urinary system assessment.

Physical Examination

Discuss the steps before beginning, reassuring the patient that the assessment should not be painful, although it may be uncomfortable at times. Inquire about any painful areas, making sure to assess these areas last. Encourage your patient to relax. Have the patient in a supine position, with the head on a pillow, knees bent or on a pillow, and arms at the sides. Learn to use distractions to enhance muscle relaxation, such as breathing exercises, engaging in conversation, and imaging. Remember to auscultate before percussion and palpation so as not to alter intestinal activity and bowel sounds.

A urinary system assessment includes body weight, vital signs, and related body structures. Begin by weighing the patient and comparing the result with a baseline figure. Note any gain or loss of about 2 to 3 pounds in a 24 to 48 hour period. This may represent a change in fluid status, verses body mass.

If possible, monitor the weight on a daily basis. In conjunction with daily weights, measure and compare fluid intake and output on a daily basis. This will aid in assessing fluid status and give clues to a fluid volume deficit or excess.

Next, assess the patient's vital signs. Measure the blood pressure in both arms, and with the patient lying down and sitting up. Orthostatic hypotension may indicate fluid volume depletion. Sustained severe hypotension results in diminished renal blood flow and may cause acute renal failure. Hypertension at rest may lead to renal insufficiency and can result from vascular damage caused by a primary renal disorder. Fever could indicate an acute urinary tract infection. Tachycardia with normal or slightly elevated blood pressure may suggest fluid overload. Bradycardia or dysrhythmias may indicate an electrolyte imbalance, such as potassium. Each of these may be caused by renal impairment.

Because the urinary system affects many body functions, it is important to assess other body structures for signs of renal involvement. Begin with assessing orientation to person, place, and time, along with memory, both recent and remote. In chronic, progressive renal failure there will be an accumulation of toxins and electrolyte imbalances, which may produce neurologic difficulties such as lethargy, confusion, disorientation, stupor, somnolence, coma, and convulsions.

There are several ways to assess the patient's hydration status. Inspect the mucous membranes in the mouth. Dryness along with parched, cracked lips reflects dehydration. Evaluate skin turgor by pinching the patient's skin with your thumb and index finger. If the skin does not return to its normal position immediately, suspect advanced dehydration. Sunken eyes reflect dehydration, whereas periorbital edema indicates a fluid excess. Inspect the patient's neck veins for distention, which indicates an excess in fluid. Often accompanying renal disease is edema, systemic or local.

Inspect the patient's skin for color, intactness, rashes, and infection. A yellow-tan cast may reflect retention of urochrom pigment, which normally colors urine yellow. Pallor stems from abnormal values in hemoglobin and hematocrit, which will typically decrease with renal failure. End-stage renal failure reduces erythropoietin production, which leads to a decrease in RBC production. Also, an increase in uremic toxins shortens the life span of the RBC. Note any ecchymoses and/or petechiae, which are characteristic signs of clotting abnormalities and decreased platelet adhesion that may reflect chronic renal failure.

Auscultate lung sounds for crackles that may reflect pulmonary edema. This can result from and increase in fluid status and renal failure. Inspect the abdomen for ascitis, which indicates an accumulation of fluid systemicly.

DIAGNOSTIC TESTS

Liver and Gallbladder

Alkaline phosphatase: an enzyme found in many tissues, with highest concentrations in the liver, biliary tract epithelium, and bone; important for determining liver and bone disorders; this enzyme is excreted into the blood when the liver is damaged as a result of obstruction of the biliary tract.

Total protein: proteins are constituents of muscle, enzymes, hormones, transport vehicles, hemoglobin, and several other key functional and structural entities within the body.

Albumin: approximately 60% of total protein is albumin with the rest being globulin; albumin is formed and synthesized within the liver and is therefore a measure of hepatocyte function; with disease, the hepatocyte loses its ability to synthesize albumin, therefore the serum albumin level is decreased.

Bilirubin: resulting from the breakdown of hemoglobin in the red blood cells, bilirubin is a by-product of hemolysis (red blood cell destruction); produced by the reticuloendothelial system and removed from the body by the liver, which excretes it into the bile; an increase may indicate excessive destruction of red blood cells, liver dysfunction or biliary obstruction.

Cholesterol: used by the body to form steroid hormones, bile acids, and most cell membranes; main use of testing is to detect disorders of blood lipids and to evaluate the risk potential for atherosclerosis related to coronary artery disease; since the liver metabolizes the cholesterol to its free form, this test may be used to aid in the study of liver function.

Alanine aminotransferase (ALT) (formerly serum glutamic-pyruvic transaminase [SGPT]): found primarily in the liver, whereas lesser quantities are found in the kidneys, heart, and skeletal muscle. Injury or disease affecting the liver or biliary obstruction will cause a release of this enzyme into the blood.

Aspartate aminotransferase (AST) (formerly serum glutamic-oxaloacetic transaminase [SGOT]): found in very high concentrations within the heart muscle, liver cells, skeletal muscle cells, and to a lesser degree, in the kidneys and pancreas; diseases that affect the hepatocyte will cause elevated levels of the enzyme in the blood.

Gamma glutamyl transpeptidase (GGT): found in highest concentrations within the liver, kidney, spleen and prostate gland; used to detect liver cell dysfunction and to detect alcohol-induced liver disease.

Urine Tests

Bilirubin: aids in the diagnosis of hepatitis and liver dysfunction; helpful in monitoring the course of treatment; bilirubin in the urine is an early sign of hepatocellular disease or biliary obstruction.

Urobilinogen: determines impaired liver function; urobilinogen is formed in the intestine; a portion of it is excreted with the feces, whereas the other portion is absorbed into the bloodstream and carried to the liver. Here it is metabolized and excreted in the bile. With an impaired liver, traces of urobilinogen escape removal from the blood by the liver and are excreted in the urine.

Liver biopsy: percutaneous liver biopsy is used in evaluating the status of the liver and diagnosing various disorders, such as cirrhosis, hepatitis, drug reaction, granuloma, and tumor.

Liver scan: used to evaluate the function, anatomy, and size of the liver.

Ultrasonography: used to determine the cystic, solid, or complex nature of a liver defect; helpful in evaluating ascitis and differentiating cysts and abscesses from tumors; also examines the gallbladder and biliary system aiding in the diagnosis of cholelithiasis and cholecystitis.

CT scan: a computer-assisted cross-sectional X-ray; used to detect disorders of the biliary tract, liver, and pancreatic disorders.

HIDA scan: a recent procedure that allows for the evaluation of hepatobiliary function; patient receives an injection of a radioactive material; a camera is used to monitor the progress of the material through the liver, bile ducts, gallbladder, and duodenum.

Oral cholecystography: allows study of the gallbladder to detect gallstones or to diagnose inflammatory disease or tumors.

Kidney

Creatinine: measures the amount of creatinine in the blood; creatinine is a by-product in the breakdown of muscle creatine phosphate resulting from energy metabolism; produced at a constant rate depending on the muscle mass of the person. Since it is then removed by the kidneys, impaired renal function would cause an increase in the blood levels; an increased creatinine level may indicate a reduction of muscle mass (malnutrition) or impaired renal function.

Blood urea nitrogen (BUN): used to assess glomerular function and the production and excretion of urea; urea is formed in the liver and constitutes the major nonprotein nitrogenous end product of protein catabolism; is then removed by the kidneys; an increase in BUN may indicate an impairment in kidney function.

Uric acid: the end product of purine metabolism; two thirds are excreted by the kidneys and one third by the intestines; test can be used to evaluate kidney function.

Urinalysis (UA): analysis of the urine is used to identify abnormal constituents; abnormal levels and the presence of some constituents indicate the possibility of abnormalities in the glomerular membrane, infection or trauma.

Kidney-ureter-bladder x-ray (KUB): an anteroposterior x-ray of the kidneys, ureters, and bony pelvis.

Intravenous urogram/pyelogram (IVU / IVP): a series of contrast-enhanced radiographic x-rays that allows visualization of the size, shape, and structure of kidneys, ureters, and bladder and the ability of the bladder to empty sufficiently; kidney disease, ureteral or bladder stones, and tumors can be detected with this test.

Retrograde pyelogram (RPG): consists of a series of x-rays that provide detailed information of the upper urinary tract (ureter, ureteropelvic junction, renal pelvis, and calyces) using cystoscopy to introduce catheters into the ureters where iodine contrast dye will be injected.

Renal arteriogram: a series of x-rays that allows detailed evaluation of the arterial supply of the kidneys.

Renal computed tomography (CT Scan): provides computer-generated axial images of the abdominal contents, including the kidneys, ureters, bladder, and major renal vessels; it is used to detect renal masses, lesions, and enlarged lymph nodes resulting from metastatic invasion.

Radionuclide imaging (renal scan): provides computer images of urinary tract structures. They are used to evaluate the function of the urinary tract.

Kidney sonogram: uses sound waves to provide an image of the urinary system organs, including the kidneys, ureters, and bladder. Hydronephrosis, dilated ureters, calculi solid tumors, and cysts can be detected.

Pancreas

Amylase

Amylase is an enzyme that is produced in the salivary glands, pancreas, liver, and fallopian tubes. It is used to change starch to sugar. This test can be used to detect inflammation of the pancreas or salivary glands.

Lipase

Lipase is an enzyme secreted by the pancreas into the duodenum to break down triglycerides into fatty acids. This test is used to evaluate the function of the pancreas.

Gastrointestinal

Electrolytes: tests provide a quantitative analysis of major intracellular and extracellular electrolytes.

Calcium: Increased level: metabolic alkalosis
  Decreased level: malabsorption, alkalosis, diarrhea

Sodium: Increased level: dehydration; diarrhea
  Decreased level: diarrhea, vomiting, pyloric obstruction, malabsorption, excessive stomach drainage

Chloride: Increased level: dehydration
  Decreased level: vomiting, diarrhea, pyloric obstruction

Bicarbonate: Increased level: metabolic alkalosis caused by loss of gastric acids from vomiting or gastric drainage
  Decreased level: metabolic acidosis caused by persistent diarrhea

Phosphate: Increased level: high intestinal obstruction
  Decreased level: malnutrition, malabsorption

Potassium: Decreased level: diarrhea, pyloric obstruction, malabsorption, vomiting, starvation,

Magnesium: Increased level: dehydration
  Decreased level: malabsorption, prolonged gastric drainage, diarrhea

Barium swallow (upper GI series): used to examine the esophagus, stomach, duodenum, and upper part of the jejunum; contrast medium is used along with fluoroscopy to examine the position, patency, and contour of the above structures.

Barium enema (lower GI series): allows for the examination of the colon; used to detect the presence and location of inflammatory disorders, polyps, tumors, and diverticula.

Angiography: with the use of a radiographic contrast, examines the vascular system; used to determine the site of gastrointestinal bleeding and to detect ischemia and angiodysplasia.

Endoscopy: uses a fiberoptic endoscope that is passed through the patient's mouth and into his esophagus, stomach, and duodenum; or is passed through his anus and into his large intestine.

> **Esophagogastroduodenoscopy**: allows the visualization of the esophageal, stomach, and upper duodenal lining; used to detect inflammation, ulcers, varices, strictures, hiatal hernias, mucosal lesions, and carcinoma.

> **Proctosigmoidoscopy**: provides visualization of the distal sigmoid colon, the rectum, and the anal canal; used to detect hemorrhoids, polyps, fissures, fistulas, abscesses, and inflammatory, infectious, and/or ulcerative bowel diseases.

> **Colonscopy**: provides visualization of the lining of the large intestine; used to diagnose inflammatory and ulcerative bowel disease and colonic strictures and lesions to locate the origin of lower gastrointestinal bleeding and to assess for recurring polyps or malignant lesions.

Small bowel biopsy: examines the mucosa of the small bowel for malabsorption disorders.

NURSING DIAGNOSES

Altered Urinary Elimination

Definition: the state in which an individual experiences or is at risk of experiencing a change in urinary function.

Related Factors
- Anatomical obstruction
- Sensory motor impairment
- Neuromuscular impairment
- Urinary tract infection
- Mechanical trauma
- Dehydration
- Decreased attention to bladder cues (depression, sedation, confusion)
- Fear
- Stress
- Effects of aging, medications, pregnancy, surgery
- Immobility
- Indwelling catheter
- Lack of privacy
- Prolonged bed rest

Defining Characteristics
Subjective: verbal reports of frequency, hesitancy, dysuria, urgency.
Objective: nocturia, urgency, incontinence, retention, distended bladder.

Urinary retention

Definition: The state in which an individual experiences incomplete emptying of the bladder.

Related Factors

- Diminished or absent sensory and/or motor impulses
- Effects of medications (anesthetics, opiates, psychotropics, antihistamines, atropine, belladonna)
- Anxiety
- High urethral pressure caused by weak detrusor
- Strong sphincter
- Urethral blockage associated with:
  Fecal impaction
  Postpartum edema
  Prostate hypertrophy
  Surgical swelling
- Inhibition of reflex arc

Defining Characteristics

Subjective: verbal reports of sensation of bladder fullness, dribbling, dysuria.
Objective: bladder distention, diminished force of urinary stream; dribbling; small, frequent voiding or absence of urine output.

Stress incontinence

Definition: the state in which an individual experiences an involuntary passage of urine of less than 50 ml accompanied by increased abdominal pressure.

Related Factors

- Degenerative changes in pelvic muscles and structural supports associated with increased age
- High intraabdominal pressure (obesity, pregnancy)
- Incompetent bladder outlet
- Overdistention between voidings
- Weak pelvic muscles and structural supports

Defining Characteristics

Subjective: verbal reports of reported dribbling with increased abdominal pressure (coughing, sneezing, lifting, aerobics, changing positions); urgency
Objective: urgency; frequency (more than every 2 hours); loss of urine in standing position; observed dribbling associated with increased abdominal pressure

Reflex incontinence

Definition: the state in which an individual experiences an involuntary passage of urine occurring at predictable intervals when a specific bladder volume is reached.

Related Factors
- Neurologic impairment such as spinal cord injury or tumor

Defining Characteristics
Subjective: verbal reports of no awareness of being incontinent; no awareness of bladder filling; no urge to void or feelings of fullness.
Objective: voids in large amounts; uninhibited bladder contraction/spasm at regular intervals; somewhat predictable voiding pattern.

Urge incontinence

Definition: the state in which an individual experiences involuntary passage of urine occurring soon after a strong sense of urgency to void.

Related Factors
- Bladder infection/irritation
- Changes in urine concentration
- Decreased bladder capacity associated with:
  - Abdominal surgeries
  - History of pelvic inflammatory disease
  - Indwelling catheter
- Overdistention of bladder
- Diuretic therapy
- Ingestion of alcohol, caffeine, or increased fluids

Defining Characteristics
Subjective: verbal reports of urinary urgency; frequency (more often than every 2 hours); bladder contracture/spasm; nocturia (more than 2 times per night).
Objective: nocturia; urgency; frequency; inability to reach toilet in time; voiding in small amounts (less than 100 ml) or in large amounts (more than 550 ml)

Functional incontinence

Definition: the state in which an individual experiences involuntary and unpredictable passage of urine.

Related Factors

- Altered environment
- Cognitive/sensory deficits (inattentiveness to urge to void, use of sedation)
- Mobility deficits (difficulty in removing clothes)
- Increased urine production
- Reluctance to use call light or bedpan

Defining Characteristics

Subjective: verbal reports of urge to void or bladder contractions sufficiently strong to result in loss of urine before reaching an appropriate receptacle; unrecognized signals of bladder fullness; unpredictable voiding pattern.
Objective: voiding in large amounts.

Total incontinence

Definition: the state in which an individual experiences a continuous and unpredictable passage of urine

Related Factors

- Neurological dysfunction causing triggering of micturation at unpredictable times
- Neuromuscular trauma related to surgical procedures
- Neuropathy preventing transmission of reflex indicating bladder fullness
- Fistulas secondary to trauma
- Trauma or disease affecting spinal cord/nerves

Defining Characteristics

Subjective: verbal reports of constant flow of urine occurs at unpredictable times without distention; incontinence refractory to therapy; nocturia; lack of perineal or bladder filling awareness; unawareness of incontinence; inhibited bladder contractions/spasms.
Objective: unsuccessful incontinence refractory treatments.

Bowel incontinence

Definition: the state in which an individual experiences an inability to control the passage of bowel movements.

Related Factors

- Diarrhea
- Fecal impaction
- Impairment: cognitive, neuromuscular, perceptual
- Effects of medications
- Excessive use of laxatives
- Depression
- Anxiety
- Loss of sphincter control

Defining Characteristics

Subjective: verbal reports of urgency; lack of awareness of need to defecate; lack of awareness of passage of stool.
Objective: involuntary passage of stool; rectal oozing of stool.

Diarrhea

Definition: the state in which the individual experiences or is at risk of experiencing a change in normal bowel movements resulting in frequent, loose, or liquid stools.

Related Factors

- Effects of medications, radiation, surgical intervention
- Side effects of antibiotics
- Excessive use of laxatives
- Allergies
- Inflammatory process
- Infectious process
- Malabsorption syndrome
- Nutritional disorders
- Stress and anxiety
- Dietary alterations: food intolerances, high cellulose foods, increased caffeine consumption, hyperosmolar tube feeding
- Ingestion of contaminated water or food

Defining Characteristics

Subjective: verbal reports of abdominal pain; urgency; cramping; anorexia; chills; fatigue; irritated anal area; malaise; thirst; increased frequency of stools.
Objective: increased frequency of stools; increased frequency of bowel sounds; loose, liquid stools; change in color or odor of stool; fever; mucoid stool; weight loss.

Fluid volume excess

Definition: the state in which an individual experiences or is at risk for experiencing an excess of body fluids.

Related Factors

- Compromised regulatory mechanisms (aldosterone, antidiuretic hormone, renin-angiotensin)
- Excessive fluid or sodium intake
- Low protein intake (e.g. malnutrition, draining fistulas, burns, organ failure)
- Effects of medications (e.g. chlorpropamide, tolbutamide, vincristine, triptyline, carbamazepine)
- Effects of age
- Effects of pregnancy

Defining Characteristics

Subjective: Verbal reports of dyspnea; orthopnea; anxiety

Objective: dyspnea; abnormal breath sounds (rales); pulmonary congestion; change in respiratory pattern; azotemia, altered electrolytes; edema; effusions; anasarca; weight gain; intake greater than output; third heart sound (S3); change in mental status; restlessness; blood pressure changes; central venous distention; positive hepatojugular reflex; oliguria; specific gravity changes; decreased hemoglobin, hematocrit; muscular twitching/weakness; nausea and/or vomiting.

Fluid volume deficit (actual or potential)

Deficit #1 - regulatory failure

Definition: the state in which an individual experiences vascular, cellular, or intracellular dehydration (in excess of needs or replacement capabilities caused by failure of regulatory mechanisms)

Related Factors

- Failure of regulatory mechanisms
- Extremes of age
- Fever
- Fluid shift to extravascular space
- Increased metabolic rate
- Infection

Defining Characteristics

Subjective: verbal reports of fatigue; nervousness; thirst; weakness.

Objective: increased urine output; dilute urine; sudden weight loss; decreased venous filling; hemoconcentration; altered serum sodium; decreased blood pressure; decreased pulse volume/pressure; dry skin and mucous membranes; poor skin turgor, edema; increased pule rate; increased body temperature; thirst, weakness.

Fluid volume deficit (actual or potential)

Deficit #2 - active loss

Definition: the state in which an individual experiences vascular, cellular, or intracellular dehydration (in excess of needs or replacement capabilities due to active loss).

Related Factors

- Loss of body fluids or electrolytes
- Diaphoresis
- Difficulty swallowing, eating
- Excessive drainage through artificial orifices or lumens, wounds, or drainage tubes
- Imposed fluid restriction
- Hyperventilation
- Increased insensible water loss
- Nausea and/or vomiting
- Climate exposure (extreme heat)
- Dietary alterations
- Diuretic therapy
- Excessive use of alcohol, enemas, laxatives

Defining Characteristics

Subjective: verbal reports of thirst; weakness.

Objective: decreased urine output; output greater than intake; decreased venous filling; increased serum sodium; concentrated urine; sudden weight loss; hemoconcentration; change in mental status, decreased blood pressure, decreased pulse volume/pressure; poor skin turgor; dry skin and mucous membranes; increased body temperature; increased pule rate; sunken eyeballs; thirst; weakness.

Altered tissue perfusion (renal, gastrointestinal)

Definition: the state in which an individual experiences a decrease in nutrition or oxygenation at the cellular level because of a deficit in capillary blood supply.

Related Factors

- Interruption of arterial flow
- Interruption of venous flow
- Hypervolemia
- Hypovolemia
- Trauma
- Prolonged sitting/standing
- Immobilization
- Oxygen/carbon dioxide exchange problems
- Decreased cardiac output
- Increased peripheral vascular resistance

Defining Characteristics

Subjective

Renal: verbal reports of decreased urinary output, weight gain

Gastrointestinal: verbal reports of alteration in bowel movement pattern, nausea, vomiting, decreased appetite

Objective

Renal: decreased urine output, edema, increased specific gravity, increased BUN, hematuria confusion, blurred vision, syncope/vertigo, unequal or dilated pupils

Gastrointestinal: vomiting, abdominal distention, constipation, melena

Related Nursing Diagnoses
Anxiety
Constipation
Colonic constipation
Perceived constipation
Fatigue
Altered Nutrition (more than body requirements)
Altered Nutrition (less than body requirements)

CASE STUDY

Mr. K. is a 47-year-old male who came into the emergency room with complaints of severe abdominal pain and blood in his stool.

Health History

Chief complaint: severe abdominal pain

Present problem: reports intermittent bouts of diarrhea for 3 months since his divorce (approximately 7-10 stools per day) along with fatigue; has been using over-the-counter anti-diarrhea medications with temporary relief; patient states he has been losing weight since the diarrhea began; verbalizes a decrease in appetite; has been experiencing some abdominal discomfort for approximately 4 days but first noted blood in the stool yesterday; early this A.M. abdominal pain intensified and decided to come to the emergency room.

Past medical history: depression

Family History: mother and father alive and well

Social History: smokes 1 1/2 packs/day x 20 years; use of alcohol 3-4 x weekly in social setting; was divorced 3 months before admission dissolving a 22 year marriage; verbalizes fear and anxiety concerning being single again and living on one income.

Physical Examination

General: 47-year-old male: ht 5'11", wt 154 lb, BP 122/86, pulse 82, resp 20, temp 97.7° F.

Inspection: abdomen flat without scars or masses; no pulsations or peristalsis visible.

Auscultation: hyperactive bowel sounds heard in all quadrants

Percussion: tympany in all four quadrants; liver span 8 cm at right midclavicular line

Palpation: tenderness in all four quadrants (facial grimacing and guarding); no organomegaly, no liver tenderness; spleen not palpable; no costovertebral angle tenderness.

Problems identified for Mr. K.

Pain related to irritation of the gastric mucosa

Defining Characteristics

Subjective: complain of abdominal pain.

Objective: grimacing of face when abdomen is palpated; guarding behavior of entire abdomen.

Diarrhea related to irritation of gastric mucosa

Defining Characteristics

Subjective: verbalizes 7 to 10 stools per day; takes over-the-counter anti-diarrhea medication; abdominal pain; cramping.

Objective: 7 to 10 stools per day; increased frequency of bowel sounds; abdominal tenderness upon palpation.

Altered nutrition: less than body requirement related to abdominal pain and decreased appetite

Defining Characteristics

Subjective: verbalizes a decrease in appetite; abdominal pain.

Objective: recent weight loss.

High risk for fluid volume deficit (active loss) related to diarrhea

Defining Characteristics

Subjective: decreased appetite; 7 to 10 stools per day; fatigue.

Objective: 7 to 10 stools per day; hyperactive bowel sounds.

Anxiety related to situational crisis (recent divorce)

Defining Characteristics

Subjective: verbalizes fear and anxiety about being single again and living on one income.

Objective: recent divorce; history of depression.

HEALTH PROMOTION

Preventing urinary tract infections

- Practice good hygiene
- Women wipe from front to back after defecation
- Showering/bathing daily cleansing perineal area thoroughly
- Avoid perfume sprays
- Avoid bubble baths and perfumed oils
- Wash perineal area after using spermicidal jelly or foam
- Drink plenty of fluids
- Drink 2 to 4 liters per day
- Avoid excessive intake of carbonated beverages, coffee, tea, and alcoholic drinks
- Urinate on a regular basis, drink waking hours (every 2-4 hours as needed)
- Seek professional help if you think you might have a urinary bladder infection

Signs of urinary tract infection

- Frequent and urgent need to urinate
- Pain in the lower back and lower pelvic region
- Cloudy or foul-smelling urine
- Bloody urine
- Chills or fever
- Lack of appetite and/or lack of energy

Ways to avoid an ulcer

- Use acetaminophen (Tylenol) or buffered aspirin for pain relief
- Eat three balanced meals a day
- Avoid any foods that cause gastric discomfort
- Avoid hot and spicy foods
- If alcohol is taken drink minimally and not on an empty stomach
- Avoid stress at mealtimes and plan for a quiet time after eating
- Stop smoking if possible
- Participate in recreation and hobbies that promote relaxation
- Provide for a good night's sleep on a regular basis
- Structure home and work environment to keep stressors at a reasonable level

Female Genitalia

NURSING CONSIDERATIONS

Health History

Assessment of the genitalia involves much more than mere anatomy and physiology. It involves the concept of human sexuality, which makes this topic more emotional and complex. Sexuality refers to a person's perceptions, thoughts, feelings, and behaviors related to sexual identity and sexual interaction with others. Often reproductive development and function affect an individual's perception of one's own sexuality. In the past and still somewhat today, the patient's sexual and reproductive functions are omitted from the health history. Only recently have health care professionals recognized the relevance of sexual health as a component of well-being. There are so many aspects that affect sexual function and satisfaction, such as illnesses, surgical procedures, physiologic aging processes, and medications, that it is vital that we include sexual health as a part of every health history. The health history provides an opportunity to evaluate the patient's understanding of sexual and reproductive function and identify teaching needs.

It is not always an easy process to include this information in the health history. There may be many barriers to obtaining accurate data. Sex or sexual function has long been considered an inappropriate topic for conversation. We often encounter cultural taboos in not only discussing sexual matters but also in permitting the physical examination of a female patient. It is important that the interviewer provide detailed information and explanations about why such confidential information is necessary.

Another barrier may be terminology and language. The interviewer must find a common ground for understanding. This means that we need to be certain about what the patient's statements mean and use terms that the patient understands. Derogatory or judgmental terms should be avoided. More importantly, do not allow personal prejudices to develop toward the patient and do not inject your own values, morals, or beliefs into the discussion. It is also necessary to be aware of and acknowledge your own beliefs, feelings, comfort levels, and limitations in discussing sexuality and sexual functioning. We need to convey a professional attitude about the importance of sexual function in health promotion by making every effort to understand the views, perceptions, and language of the patient.

Incorporate questions about sexuality into the initial interview in a routine manner. Make sure the environment is comfortable and private. To ensure patient comfort and confidence, the interview should be unhurried with the patient seated and dressed.

Physical Examination

The physical examination is important in evaluating the cause of sexual concerns or problems and may be the best opportunity to teach the patient about sexuality. Women often have negative feelings and/or feel anxious about the pelvic assessment because of cultural or personal beliefs or the mere discomfort of the examination. The examiner needs to be aware of these feelings and concerns and to reassure the woman by offering support and guidance and to provide a warm, friendly atmosphere. Explain the procedure and answer all questions before the woman is placed in the lithotomy position so she may anticipate what will happen and thereby maintain a sense of personal control. Offer the patient a mirror so she can view her genitals as you explain anatomy, physiology, and the procedure. Some women may not wish to view the assessment; you should respect their decision.

DIAGNOSTIC TESTS

Gynecological examination: consists of 2 parts: (1) Papanicolaou smear (pap smear), and (2) pelvic examination.

The Pap smear is one of the most effective ways to detect cancers of the cervix in its earliest and most curable stages. During the Pap smear, a speculum is inserted into the vagina so the cervix and vaginal walls can be directly examined. A small scraping of cells is taken from the cervix and placed on a microscopic slide. In this test, abnormal cells can be identified with a microscope before outward signs appear. Smears for cancer and cultures for sexually transmitted diseases can be taken from several areas: endocervix, cervix, vagina, anal, and oropharyngeal.

During the pelvic examination, the examiner places two fingers in the vagina so that the uterus, vagina, ovaries and cervix can be examined and assessed for any abnormality in size or shape.

NURSING DIAGNOSES

Body image disturbance

Definition: the state in which an individual experiences a negative or distorted perception of the body.

Related Factors

- Physical trauma/mutilation
- Pregnancy
- Physical change caused by biochemical agents (drugs)
- Dependence on machine
- Effects of loss of body part(s)
- Effects of loss of body function

with regard to age, sex, developmental level or basic human needs
- Psychosocial difficulties
- Cultural or spiritual difficulties
- Maturational changes

Defining Characteristics

Subjective: verbal reports of change in lifestyle; fear of rejection or reaction by others; preoccupation with change or loss; feelings of helplessness, hopelessness, or powerlessness; refusal to verify actual change; refusal to participate in self-care; negative feelings about self; focuses on past strength, function, or appearance; guilt or shame.

Objective: missing body part; actual change in structure and/or function; hiding or overexposing body part; trauma to nonfunctioning part; change in ability to estimate spatial relationship of body to environment; extension of body boundary to incorporate environmental objects; preoccupation with change or loss; change in social involvement; not looking at or touching body part.

Ineffective individual coping

Definition: the state in which an individual demonstrates impaired adaptive behaviors and problem-solving abilities.

Related Factors

- Situational crises
- Maturational crises
- Personal vulnerability
- Inadequate coping skills
- Unrealistic perceptions
- Multiple stressors/life changes
- Major changes in lifestyle
- Inadequate relaxation/leisure activities
- Low self-esteem
- Unmet expectations
- Poor nutrition
- Work overload
- Too many deadlines
- Unrealistic perceptions
- Inadequate support systems
- Little or no exercise
- Knowledge deficit regarding therapeutic regimen, disease process, and/or prognosis
- Sensory overload
- Severe pain
- Overwhelming threat to self
- Impairment to nervous system

Definining Characteristics

Subjective: verbal reports of inability to cope; inability too meet expectations; inability to ask for help; inability to problem solve; verbal manipulation, reports of chronic worry/anxiety/depression; lack of appetite; chronic fatigue; insomnia; general irritability.

Objective: insomnia; physical inactivity; substance abuse; alteration in societal participation, destructive behavior toward self or others; inappropriate use of defense mechanisms; change in usual communication patterns; inability to meet or take responsibility for basic needs; exaggerated fear of pain, death; general irritability; high rate of injuries or illnesses; frequent headaches/neckaches; indecisiveness, overeating; excessive smoking; excessive drinking; irritable bowel, poor self-esteem; lack of assertive behaviors.

Sexual dysfunction

Definition: the state in which an individual's sexual health or function is viewed as unrewarding or inadequate.

Related Factors

- Ineffectual or absent role models
- Disturbance in self-esteem or body image
- Lack of significant other
- Physical abuse
- Psychosocial abuse
- Values conflict
- Vulnerability
- Misinformation or lack of knowledge
- Lack of privacy
- Altered body structure or function: pregnancy, recent childbirth, drugs, surgery, disease process, trauma, loss of sexual desire
- Change in interest in self and/or others
- Alterations in achieving perceived sex role or sexual satisfaction

Defining Characteristics

Subjective: verbal reports of problem in sexuality; actual or perceived limitation imposed by disease and/or therapy; inability to achieve desired satisfaction; conflicts involving values; alterations in achieving sexual satisfaction; seeking confirmation of desirability; alteration in relationship with significant other; change in interest in self and/or others.

Objective: alteration in relationship with significant other; change of interest in self and others; impotence, delayed development of secondary sexual characteristics; exhibitionism; voyeurism; guilt; masochism/sadism; sexual promiscuity.

Anxiety

Definition: a vague uneasy feeling, the source of which is often nonspecific or unknown to the individual.

Related Factors

- Threat to self-concept
- Situational and/or maturational crisis
- Interpersonal transmission and contagion
- Threat of death (perceived or actual)
- Threat to or change in health status
- Threat to or change in role functioning
- Threat to or change in environment
- Threat to or change in interaction patterns
- Threat to or change in socioeconomic status
- Unmet needs
- Unconscious conflict about essential values and goals of life

Defining Characteristics

Subjective: verbal reports of increased tension; apprehension; uncertainty; feeling of being scared; feeling of inadequacy; shakiness; fear of unspecified consequences; overexcitedness; increased helplessness; regretfulness; feeling of being rattled; distress; jitteriness.

Objective: sympathetic stimulation - cardiovascular excitation, superficial vasoconstriction, pupil dilation; restlessness; insomnia; glancing about; poor eye contact; trembling; hand tremors; extraneous movements - footshuffling, hand and/or arm movements; worry; anxiety; facial tension; voice quivering; focus on self-increased wariness; increased perspiration.

Knowledge deficit (specify)

Definition: the state in which specific knowledge or skills are lacking that affect ability to maintain health.

Related Factors

- Lack of exposure or recall
- Information misinterpretation
- Unfamiliarity with information resources
- Lack of recall
- Cognitive limitations
- Lack of interest in learning
- Effects of aging
- Sensory deficits
- Language barrier
- Denial
- Inadequate economic resources

Defining Characteristics

Subjective: verbalizes the problem; repeatedly requests information; verbalizes misconception of problem.

Objective: failure to seek help or follow therapeutic regimen; inadequate performance of test; inaccurate use of health-related vocabulary; inability to explain therapeutic regimen or describe personal health status; failure to take medication; inappropriate or exaggerated behaviors, e.g., hysteria, hostility, apathy, agitation, depression.

Pain

Definition: the state in which an individual experiences and reports the presence of severe discomfort or an uncomfortable sensation.

Related Factors

- Inflammatory process
- Muscle spasm
- Effects of trauma/surgery
- Immobility
- Pressure
- Infectious process
- Overactivity
- Ischemia
- Injuring agents (biological, chemical, physical, psychological)

Defining Characteristics

Subjective: verbal reports of pain, discomfort, anxiety, uncomfortable sensation.

Objective: guarding; limping; facial mask or grimace; increased respirations; increased heart rate; increased blood pressure; anxious; restlessness; nausea; vomiting; diaphoresis; moaning; crying; pacing; self focusing.

Related Nursing Diagnoses

Self-esteem disturbance
High risk for infection
Altered role performance
Altered family processes
Altered sexuality patterns
Personal identity disturbance
Rape trauma syndrome
Powerlessness

Case Study

G.K. is a 27-year-old single female with complaints of a white, thick vaginal discharge of 10 days duration.

Health History

Chief complaint: "complains of a white, thick vaginal discharge for the last 10 days."

Present problem: approximately 10 days ago began having a white, thick vaginal discharge with no odor; this is accompanied by vaginal itching and painful intercourse; has tried several over-the-counter (OTC) medications without relief.

Past medical history: several vaginal infections in last 2 years.

Family history: mother and father alive and well.

Social history: Menarche at 13 years of age; cycle every 29 days; duration 5-6 days; mild cramps day 13 of cycle; began sexual activity at age 15; engaging in intercourse frequently with several partners; uses oral contraceptives; denies use of condoms, states "there is no need for them because I know all of my boyfriends are clean;" verbalizes some knowledge of STDs and AIDS, states "I won't get AIDS because I don't date drug users and I don't pick them up in bars."

Physical Examination

General: 27-year-old female; ht 5'6", wt 124 lb, BP 108/68, pulse 70, resp 20, temp 98.2° F.

Inspection: external genitalia is erythematous and edematous; thick, white exudate noted around introitis; vagina and cervix also erythematous and edematous with a thick, white, curdlike discharge noted on internal surfaces.

Palpation: external and internal surfaces tender to touch; no masses noted.

Diagnostic Tests

Pelvic examination and PAP smear: reveals *Candida albicans*.

Problems identified for G.K.

Pain related to vaginal tenderness and itching

Defining Characteristics

Subjective: verbalizes pain during intercourse; complains of vaginal itching.

Objective: external and internal surfaces erythematous, edematous, and tender to touch.

Sexual dysfunction related to painful intercourse

Defining Characteristics

Subjective: verbalizes pain during intercourse; complains of vaginal itching

Objective: external and internal surfaces erythematous, edematous and tender to touch

Knowledge deficit related to STDs and AIDS transmission, use of condoms

Defining Characteristics

Subjective: verbalizes some knowledge of STDs and AIDS; denies use and need of condoms; has several misconceptions concerning AIDS and the population at risk.

Objective: engages in intercourse frequently with several partners; began sexual activity at an early age; past history of several vaginal infections in past 2 years.

Other problems to consider for G.K.:

High risk for infection

Denial

HEALTH PROMOTION

Preventing infections of the genitalia
- Avoid excessive douching
- Utilize good hygiene practices
- Wash hands frequently
- Wash hands after urinating and defecating
- Daily washing or showering with soap and water
- Utilize good laundry practices
- Avoid fecal contamination by wiping the perineal area from front to back
- Avoid sexual activity with an infected partner
- Wear cotton versus nylon underwear
- Avoid tight fitting pants
- Avoid bath oils and perfume sprays
- Be aware that oral contraceptives, antibiotics and steroids increase risk of infection
- Have knowledge of the signs and symptoms of infection and seek medical assistance immediately

Detecting abnormalities of the genitalia
- Perform regular self-examination of genitalia
- Seek professional help if any changes are detected
- Routine pap smears

Male Genitalia

NURSING CONSIDERATIONS

Health History

Testicular turmors are one of the most common cancers occuring in young men today. With this in mind, all male patients should be instructed as to the importance of a genital self-examination as well as a regular, routine examination by a health professional. The majority of testicular cancers are detected by the patient or his sexual partner. Nurses should include knowledge about testicular cancer in assessment of all adolescent and adult male patients and include genital self-examination in patient teaching. The health history and physical examination provide a great opportunity to obtain information concerning the patient's knowledge and technique of the genital self-examination.

It will require tact and sensitivity when interviewing a male patient about his reproductive system. The initial goal should be to establish a rapport with the patient so he will relax and confide. One area of particular sensitivity is in the area of sexual performance. Many men associate their sexual and reproductive ability with their identities as men. Therefore, they may view problems in this area as a weakness or a sign of diminished masculinity. Older men may view a decreased sexual ability as a sign of lost youth and declining health.

Keep in mind that each patient has his own views on sexuality and reproduction, many of which may reflect cultural and religious background. During the interview, take these views into consideration and remain nonjudgmental and supportive. Throughout the interview, use terminology that is familiar and that the patient can understand; however, certain slang words may project an undesirable image of informality and intimacy.

Begin your interview by asking general questions relating to your patient's overall health of the reproductive system. As the rapport develops and your patient becomes more relaxed, then proceed to the more sensitive areas, reserving questions about sexual function until the end.

Physical Examination

The assessment of this area involves exposure and handling of the genitals, and the patient may feel anxious and embarrassed. Explain each step of the assessment process before performing it and expose only the necessary areas. It is important that the nurse feel at ease and portray a calm, professional demeanor to assist the patient in feeling comfortable during the examination. If the nurse is uncomfortable, the patient will sense this and be uncomfortable also.

DIAGNOSTIC TESTS

Syphilis Detection Tests
     Serologic test for syphilis (STS)
     Veneral disease research laboratory (VDRL)
     Rapid plasma reagin (RPR)
     Fluorescent treponemal antibody test (FTA)

The serologic tests for syphilis are used to detect antibodies to *Treponema pallidum*, the causative agent of syphilis.

Scrotal scan testicular imaging: performed on an emergency basis in the evaluation of acute painful testicular swelling; aids in the diagnosis of acute epididymitis and evaluation of injury, trauma, tumors, and masses.

NURSING DIAGNOSES

Fear

Definition: the state in which the individual experiences feelings of dread related to an identifiable source perceived as dangerous.

Related Factors
- Sensory impairment, deprivation, or overload
- Pain
- Effects of loss of body part or function
- Effects of chronic disabling illness
- Language barrier
- Threat of death, acutal or perceived
- Anticipation of events posing a threat to self-esteem
- Phobias
- Feelings of failure
- Knowledge deficit
- Learned response, conditioning
- Loss of significant other
- Separation from support system

Defining Characteristics
Subjective: verbal reports of increased tension, apprehension, impulsiveness, decreased self-assurance, fear, panic, jitteriness, nausea, "heart beating fast," feelings of loss of control.
Objective: increased alertness, concentration on source, wide-eyed, aggressive behavior, withdrawn, sympathetic stimulation: (increased heart rate, flushing, pupil dilation, vomiting, diarrhea, diaphoresis), voice tremors, urinary frequency, insomnia, increased questioning/verbalization.

Body Image Disturbance

Definition: the state in which an individual experiences a negative or distorted perception of the body.

Related Factors
- Physical trauma/mutilation
- Physical change caused by biochemical agents (drugs)
- Dependence on machine
- Effects of loss of body part(s)
- Effects of loss of body function
- with regard to age, sex, developmental level or basic human needs
- Psychosocial
- Cultural or spiritual
- Maturational changes

Defining Characteristics
Subjective: verbal reports of change in lifestyle; fear of rejection or reaction by others; preoccupation with change or loss; feelings of helplessness, hopelessness, or powerlessness; refusal to verify actual change; refusal to participate in self-care; negative feelings about self; focuses on past strength, function, or appearance; guilt or shame.

Objective: missing body part; actual change in structure and/or function; hiding or overexposing body part; trauma to nonfunctioning part; change in ability to estimate spatial relationship of body to environment; extension of body boundary to incorporate environmental objects; preoccupation with change or loss; change in social involvement; not looking at or touching body part.

Ineffective individual coping

Definition: the state in which an individual demonstrates impaired adaptive behaviors and problem-solving abilities.

Related Factors

- Situational crises
- Maturational crises
- Personal vulnerability
- Inadequate coping skills
- Unrealistic perceptions
- Multiple stressors/life changes
- Major changes in lifestyle
- Inadequate relaxation/leisure activities
- Low self-esteem
- Unmet expectations
- Poor nutrition
- Work overload
- Too many deadline
- Unrealistic perceptions
- Inadequate support systems
- Little or no exercise
- Knowledge deficit regarding therapeutic regimen, disease process and/or prognosis
- Sensory overload
- Severe pain
- Overwhelming threat to self
- Impairment to nervous system

Defining Characteristics

Subjective: verbal reports of inability to cope; inability to meet expectations; inability to ask for help; inability to problem solve; verbal manipulation, reports of chronic worry/anxiety/depression; lack of appetite; chronic fatigue; insomnia; general irritability.

Objective: insomnia; physical inactivity; substance abuse; alteration in societal participation, destructive behavior toward self or others; inappropriate use of defense mechanisms; change in usual communication patterns; inability to meet or take responsibility for basic needs; exaggerated fear of pain, death; general irritability; high rate of injuries or illnesses; frequent headaches/neckaches; indecisiveness, overeating; excessive smoking; excessive drinking; irritable bowel, poor self-esteem; lack of assertive behaviors.

Anxiety

Definition: a vague uneasy feeling, the source of which is often nonspecific or unknown to the individual.

Related Factors

- Threat to self-concept
- Situational and maturational crisis
- Interpersonal transmission and contagion
- Threat of death (perceived or actual)
- Threat to or change in health status
- Threat to or change in role functioning
- Threat to or change in environment
- Threat to or change in interaction patterns
- Threat to or change in socioeconomic status
- Unmet needs
- Unconscious conflict about essential values and goals of life

Defining Characteristics

Subjective: verbal reports of increased tension; apprehension; uncertainty; fear; feeling of being scared; feeling of inadequacy; shakiness; fear of unspecific consequences; overexcitedness; increased helplessness; regretfulness; feeling of being rattled; distress; jitteriness.

Objective: sympathetic stimulation: cardiovascular excitation, superficial vasoconstriction, pupil dilation; restlessness; insomnia; glancing about; poor eye contact; trembling; hand tremors; extraneous movements: footshuffling, hand and/or arm movements; worry; anxiety; facial tension; voice quivering; focus on self-increased wariness; increased perspiration.

Knowledge deficit (specify)

Definition: the state in which specific knowledge or skills are lacking that affect ability to maintain health.

Related Factors

- Lack of exposure or recall
- Information misinterpretation
- Unfamiliarity with information resources
- Lack of recall
- Cognitive limitations
- Lack of interest in learning
- Effects of aging
- Sensory deficits
- Language barrier
- Denial
- Inadequate economic resources

Defining Characteristics

Subjective: verbalizes the problem; repeatedly requests information; verbalizes misconception of problem.

Objective: failure to seek help or follow therapeutic regimen; inadequate performance of test; inaccurate use of health-related vocabulary; inability to explain therapeutic regimen or describe personal health status; failure to take medication; inappropriate or exaggerated behaviors, e.g., hysteria, hostility, apathy, agitation, depression.

Altered sexuality pattern

Definition: the state of changed sexual health in an individual

Related Factors

- Effects of illness or medical treatment
    - Drugs
    - Radiation
    - Anomalies
- Extreme fatigue
- Obesity
- Pain
- Performance anxiety
- Knowledge/skill deficit about alternative responses to health-related transitions
- Surgery
- Trauma
- Impaired relationship with a significant other
- Lack of significant other
- Fear of pregnancy
- Fear of acquiring a sexually transmitted disease
- Conflicts with sexual orientation or variant preferences
- Ineffective or absent role models
- Loss of job or ability to work
- Separation from or loss of significant other

Defining Characteristics

Subjective: verbal reports of difficulties, limitations or changes in sexual behaviors or activities.

Case Study

S.M. is a 21-year-old male college student who came into the clinic because of a sore on his penis.

Health History

Chief complaint: "I have a sore on my penis and I'm having difficulty urinating."

Present problem: states "about 3 weeks ago I had unprotected sex with a girl who I thought later might have been dirty. I know it was stupid, but I didn't think one time would hurt and it takes so long to put a condom on. Nobody has to know, do they?"; complains of difficulty in urination with frequency.

Past medical history: none.

Family history: non-contributory.

Social history: states that most of the time he uses a condom; also expresses concern about having sex with his present steady girlfriend.

Physical Examination

General: 21-year-old male: ht 6'0", wt 175 lb; BP 120/72, pulse 92, resp 20, temp 99.8° F.

Inspection: very anxious (wringing hands, pacing and tapping of fingers); oval indurated ulcer on penis with raised edges; urethral meatus has mild edema with small amount of thick, white drainage; no genital skin rash noted; scrotum rugated without lesions of erythema.

Palpation: penis and urethral meatus tender to touch; testes symmetrically sized with no masses noted; bilateral inquinal, nontender lymph nodes approximately 2 cm in diameter, freely moving; firm with tenderness.

Diagnostic Procedures

Serologic test: positive for syphilis

Problems identified for S.M.

Impaired skin integrity related to penile ulcer

Defining Characteristics

Subjective: verbalizes presence of sore on penis

Objective: presence of oval indurated ulcer with raised edges on penis

Knowledge deficit related to information misinterpretation.
(Lack of knowledge concerning the importance of wearing a condom consistently.)

Defining Characteristics

Subjective: verbalized it was "stupid" to have had unprotected sex; suspected that he was infected; verbalized that he thought one time would not hurt; does not consistently use condoms.

Objective: had unprotected sex with someone he thought was infected.

Altered sexuality pattern related to presence of infectious process in reproductive system.

Defining Characteristics

Subjective: expressed concern about having sex with his present steady girlfriend.

Objective: presence of sore on penis; presence of drainage from urethral meatus.

Anxiety related to infectious process in reproductive system.

Defining Characteristics

Subjective: expressed concern about other people knowing about his situation; expressed concern about having sex with his present steady girlfriend.

Objective: very anxious (wringing hands, pacing and tapping of fingers); ulcer present on penis.

Related Nursing Diagnoses
Self-esteem disturbance
High risk for infection
Ineffective family coping
Altered role performance
Altered family processes
Noncompliance
Personal identity disturbance
Hyperthermia
Impaired skin integrity
Sexual dysfunction

HEALTH PROMOTION

Preventing cancer of the testes
- Perform regular testicular self-examinations
- Seek professional help if any changes are detected

Preventing sexually transmitted diseases (STDs)
- Safest means of preventing STDs is a mutually monogamous relationship between two uninfected persons
- If not mutually monogamous, limit the number of other sexual partners
- Inquire about previous and current sexual partner
- Use a condom made of latex with a spermicide during contact: vaginal and anal intercourse, and for oral-penile contact
- High-risk activities include vaginal and anal intercourse without a condom, oral-penile contact, oral-vulvar contact, contact between a partner's semen or urine and a mucous membrane (vagina, rectum, urethra, mouth, eye), oral-anal contact, and blood contact (menstrual blood)

Anus, Rectum and Prostate

NURSING CONSIDERATIONS

Health History

Many patients consider their gastrointestinal function, especially their bowel habits, a private matter and may feel uncomfortable discussing it. It is, however, very important to explore all complaints as they may signal a serious underlying problem, even if the patient may dismiss them as unimportant. To facilitate honest and complete patient interaction on this subject, conduct the health history interview in private. Discuss all aspects of the interview and examination before beginning.

Physical Examination

It is not uncommon to find written in the patient's record that the rectal examination has been deferred. Many times it has been deferred due to cultural and sexual attitudes or problems on the part of the patient and health care worker. Pathology can occur in the genitals and rectum as easily as any other anatomic regions of the body. It then becomes important to have a positive attitude toward examination of this region. Keep in mind that physical assessment of this area is directed toward promotion of health and detection of disease. Usually, a routine rectal examimation is performed only on a patient over age 40; however, it may be performed on any patient with a history of bowel elimination changes, anal discomfort, constipation, or an adult male with a urinary problem.

DIAGNOSTIC TESTS

Stool and anal cultures and smears: commonly done to identify parasites, enteric disease organisms, and viruses in the intestinal tract.

Proctoscopy, sigmoidoscopy: involve the visualization/examination of a 25-cm area of the rectum and sigmoid with a proctosigmoidoscope; since half of all carcinomas occur in the rectum and colon, these examinations are of particular importance; the early detection of polyps and malignant lesions may result in early and successful treatment of an otherwise fatal disease.

Blood in stool: the normal person passes a very small amount of blood into the gastrointestinal tract daily; usually, this bleeding is not significant enough to cause a positive result in stool for occult (hidden) blood; detection of occult blood in the stool is very useful in detecting or localizing disease of the gastrointestinal tract; however, the real benefit is the screening for colonic carcinoma and other sources of occult bleeding.

Prostate-specific antigen (PSA) : a glycoprotein that is normally found in the cytoplasm of prostatic epithelial cells and is detected in all males; level increases in patients with prostatic cancer; the higher the levels, the greater the tumor burden. PSA levels are also useful in monitoring the response to therapy (surgery, radiation, or hormone therapy) and may indicate a recurrence of prostatic cancer.

Acid Phosphatase or Prostatic Acid Phosphatase (PAP): primarily used to diagnose and stage prostatic carcinoma; can also be used to monitor the effectiveness of treatment; elevated levels are seen in patients with prostatic cancer that has metastasized beyond the capsule to other parts of the body.

NURSING DIAGNOSES

Constipation

Definition: the state in which an individual experiences a change in normal bowel habits characterized by a decrease in frequency and/or passage of hard, dry stools.

Related Factors
- Less than adequate intake
- Less than adequate dietary intake and bulk
- Less than adequate physical activity or immobility
- Personal habits
- Medications
- Chronic use of enemas or laxatives
- Gastrointestinal obstructive lesions
- Neuromuscular impairment
- Musculoskeletal impairment
- Pain on defecation
- Diagnostic procedures
- Lack of privacy
- Weak abdominal musculature
- Pregnancy
- Emotional status

Defining Characteristics
Subjective: verbal reports of frequency less than usual pattern; reported feeling of abdominal or rectal fullness or pressure; nausea.
Objective: hard formed stools; decreased quantity; palpable mass; straining at stool; decreased activity level; decreased bowel sounds; abdominal distention.

Other possible defining characteristics include abdominal pain; back pain; headache; interference with daily living; use of laxatives; decreased appetite.

Perceived Constipation

Definition: the state in which an individual makes a self-diagnosis of constipation and ensures a daily bowel movement through use of laxatives, enemas, and suppositories.

Related Factors
- Cultural/family health beliefs
- Faulty appraisal of bowel elimination habits
- Impaired thought processes

Defining Characteristics
Subjective: verbal reports of expectation of a daily bowel movement with the resulting overuse of laxatives, enemas, and suppositories; expected passage of stool at same time every day.

Bowel Incontinence

Definition: the state in which an individual experiences a change in normal bowel habits characterized by involuntary passage of stool.

Related Factors
- Severe anxiety/stress
- Neuromuscular involvement
- Musculoskeletal involvement
- Depression
- Perceptual or cognitive impairment

Defining Characteristic
Objective: involuntary passage of stool

Case Study

Mrs. J. is a 52-year-old female complaining of itching and burning in the rectal area.

Health History

Chief complaint: burning and itching in the rectal area.

Present problem: approximately 3-4 days ago began to notice some burning and itching around the rectum especially after each bowel movement; verbalizes difficulty in passing her stool, which is hard and painful; notes a little blood on the toilet tissue after each bowel movement; states usual bowel habits consist of one movement per day; last bowel movement was 2 days ago; has been taking a laxative everyday and occasionally uses an enema.

Past medical history: hemorrhoids (since last pregnancy 20 years ago).

Social history: does very little exercise; states that she is trying to lose weight and does not eat as nutritiously as she should; a nutritonal history reveals that the diet is low in roughage, high in fat, and fluid intake of approximately 600-800ml/day.

Physical Examination

General: 52-year-old obese female: ht 5'4", wt 215 lb.

Inspection: abdomen protrudes; no pulsations or peristalsis visualized; 2 cm x 2 cm blue-red swollen mass noted below the anorectal junction; slight redness noted around rectum.

Palpation: abdomen soft without tenderness; no masses felt; rectal sphincter tone good; rectal wall smooth; verbalizes discomfort upon palpation of rectum and rectal mass; no impaction felt.

Percussion: tympany all four quadrants.

Auscultation: normal bowel sounds all four quadrants.

Diagnostic Procedures

Stool for occult blood: negative.

Problems identified for Mrs. J.

Constipation related to low roughage diet and low fluid intake

Defining Characteristics

Subjective: has not have bowel movement for 2 days; does not eat as nutritiously as she should.

Objective: frequency less than normal pattern; hard formed stools, straining at stool; bleeding; 2 cm x 2 cm mass.

Pain related to constipation

Defining Characteristics

Subjective: verbalizes pain during defecation and rectal examination;.

Objective: presence of hemorrhoids

HEALTH PROMOTION

Ways to prevent constipation

- Plan the daily schedule to allow time for defecation when it usually occurs
- Eat a high-fiber diet (whole grain cereals and breads, fresh fruits and vegetables, nuts, and seeds)
- Supplement diet with bran (in moderation)
- Drink at least 2000 ml/day (8 glasses of 240 ml each)
- Participate in daily exercise such as walking, exercises, sports
- Avoid chronic use of laxatives, if possible

Predisposing factors for hemorrhoids

- Heredity
- Long periods of standing or sitting
- Prostatic enlargement
- Chronic liver disease
- Increased intraabdominal pressure
- Constipation
- Straining at defecation
- Pregnancy

Prevention of colorectal cancer

- No primary prevention measures are known
- Secondary prevention involves early detection
- Notify physician of any change in bowel patterns such as constipation, diarrhea, change in shape of the stool, pass blood
- Regular screening by a physician:
    Digital rectal examination yearly after age 40
    Occult blood stool test yearly after age 50
    Proctosigmoidoscopy every 3-5 years after age 50, following 2 negative yearly examinations
- Recommending a high-fiber, low-fat diet (has not been established to prevent cancer)

Nursing Considerations and Nursing Diagnoses
to Accompany Chapter 17

Musculoskeletal System

NURSING CONSIDERATIONS

Health History

Obtaining a thorough and accurate patient health history is crucial to the nurse's assessment of the musculoskeletal system. To obtain a full history, explore the patient's current, past, and family health status. As the interview progresses, it is important for the nurse to clarify exactly what the patient means by certain subjective complaints. There are many terms that have separate and different definitions to the health care worker that may be interchangeable to the patient, for example, stiffness, tenderness, pain, and soreness. A patient who has lived with chronic joint pain for many years can become so used to its presence that he or she may now describe the pain as an annoying soreness. It is necessary to clarify all the terms a patient may use and obtain as much related information as you can, for example, character, associated event, precipitating factors, and radiation to other areas.

Knowledge of injuries, surgeries, and treatments provides a useful guide to physical assessment activities, particularly evaluating muscle strength and joint range-of-motion. A thorough review of possible familial tendencies towards musculoskeletal problems gives a clue to the possible conditions for which the patient may be at risk.

All the information obtained in the health history gives the nurse clues to the extent at which the patient can function and participate in the activities of daily living. The patient's personal habits, sleep and wake patterns, and typical daily activities are explored. Also, because musculoskeletal problems can profoundly affect role and relationship patterns, these areas should also be investigated.

Physical Examination

There are certain general rules that apply to the musculoskeletal examination: provide a warm, private environment; maintain respect for the patient; and uncover only what you need to see. Your approach should be unhurried and orderly. A cephalocaudal (head-to-toe), proximal-to-distal approach is recommended. As with all bilateral structures, the paired joints should be compared. During the entire examination be aware of facial expressions and body language. A patient may not verbalize pain but may do so nonverbally. Some of these cues are facial grimacing, guarding, withdrawing, and moaning.

A musculoskeletal assessment can be very tiring for the patient, especially for the elderly and the patient with compromised health. Pace the examination with frequent rest periods or schedule more than one appointment to obtain all the necessary information. Several components of the examination can be done with the patient in a sitting or lying position, which is less tiring than standing. During your evaulation of each joint range-of-motion, it may be necessary to use passive range-of-motion if the patient is too fatigued to attempt to actively move the joint.

During general inspection, the muscles are examined for gross hypertrophy or atrophy. Certain conditions may create expected changes in the muscle, for example, the athlete with hypertrophic muscles and the paralyzed patient with atrophic muscles. Both of these conditions are obvious during inspection and palpation. For the obese patient, changes in muscle mass may be difficult to assess. Although muscle mass is largely a function of the use or disuse of the muscle fibers, changes in the size of muscles may indicate disease, such as malnutrition.

Range-of-motion should be evaulated before muscle strength since the more marked muscle contraction produced with resistance may induce pain in the patient, which may skew the test results. If pain occurs during evaluation of range-of-motion, you may wish to defer further assessment of that joint. When assessing the range-of-motion of a joint there are a number of points to take into consideration:

1. A patient may voluntarily limit the motion of a joint in response to pain.
2. Spasm of the muscles involved in the movement of a joint may limit its motion.
3. Mechanical obstruction to movement may accompany bony overgrowth and scar tissue.
4. Range-of-motion may be decreased in a joint where there is inflammation of the surrounding tissues, for example, arthritis.
5. Limitation of motion in a joint may be accompanied by weakness and atrophy of the muscles that are involved.
6. Limitations in full range of motion may be an expected finding in the older patient.

As mentioned before, it is important to assess range of motion through active and passive movement. If the patient is weakened by illness, the health care worker may need to use passive movement to obtain the information. Remember, do not force a joint into a painful position. Constantly ask the patient if there is any pain and watch for facial expressions and/or nonverbal cues of pain.

For the patient who has physical limitations or imposed restrictions by equipment or the physician, you will need to use alternative methods in assessing posture. Note how the patient is sitting in the chair or lying in bed. To evaluate spinal curvature of the patient sitting in a chair, have the patient move forward slightly and assess the spine. For the patient lying in bed, position the patient in a side-lying position to observe and palpate the spine.

To assess stability and strength, you can observe the patient in a number of activities:

1. Bending over - note whether the patient bends at the waist instead of the knees; does the patient hold on to the furniture to support himself while bending and straightening?
2. Standing up from a sitting position - does the patient use his arms to push off the arms of the chair? Note whether the upper trunk leans forward before the body straightens; are the feet planted while bending and straightening?
3. Rising from a lying position - note whether the patient rolls to one side; does he push with his arms to lift up the torso; does he grab the side rails or bed side table to increase leverage?

DIAGNOSTIC TESTS

X-ray: provides information and aids in the diagnosis of musculoskeletal conditions; images obtained provide visualization of bone structures and function, which aid in detection of fractures.

Bone scan: allows the examination of the skeleton after an intravenous injection of a radionuclide material; detection of metastatic cancer to the bone is the major reason for this test, but it also is used in the evaluation of unexplained bone pain, arthritis, osteomyelitis, fractures, and abnormal healing of fractures.

Magnetic resonance imaging (MRI): provides images of body tissues that are used in the evaluation of musculoskeletal conditions, soft tissue injuries, tumors, the condition of blood vessels, and determining blood flow.

Electromyography (electromyogram): used to detect muscular disorders; electrical current is used to stimulate one or more muscle groups while the nerve and muscle response to this electrical stimulation is recorded; integrity of the nerve and muscle can be evaluated depending on the response to the stimuli.

Myelography (myelogram): uses a radiopaque solution, injected into the spinal canal, which allows visualization of the contents of the spinal canal; used to evaluate intervertebral disk integrity or herniation, the presence of tumors, or the existence of developmental or degenerative spinal conditions.

Arthrography (arthrogram): with the use of a contrast solution injected into the joint tissue, this test shows injury to ligaments, cartilage, tendons or muscles.

Arthroscopy: allows direct visualization of the interior of a joint to evaluate the condition of tissue and surrounding structures.

Alkaline phosphatase: an enzyme orginiating mainly in the bone and liver; test is used in dectecting bone disorders; in bone disease, the enzyme rises in proportion to new bone cell production.

Calcium: used by the body in processes such as muscular contraction, cardiac function, transmission of nerve impulses, and blood clotting. A patient suffering from a deficiency of ionized calcium will show signs of tetany accompanied by muscular twitching and eventual convulsions.

Rheumatoid factor (RA factor): a macroglobulin type of antibody found in the blood of persons with rheumatoid arthritis. It is believed that RF my cause or perpetuate the destructive changes associated with rheumatoid arthritis.

NURSING DIAGNOSES

Impaired physicial mobility

Definition: the state in which an individual experiences a limitation of ability for independent physical movement.

Related Factors
- Deformities
- Joint inflammation
- Bone fracture and soft tissue trauma
- Presence of restrictive devices (restraints, splint, cast,traction)
- Incorrect posture and/or alignment
- Neuromuscular impairment
- Fatigue
- Decreased strength and endurance
- Intolerance to activity
- Effects of trauma/surgery
- Pain/discomfort
- Obesity
- Side effects of sedatives/narcotics/tranquilizers
- Depression
- Severe anxiety
- Perceptual or cognitive impairment
- Architectual barriers
- Lack of assistive devices

Defining Characteristics
Subjective: verbal reports of pain, tenderness, soreness when attempting to move; stiffness; weakness; reports of no longer being able to perform usual activities and/or desired activities.
Objective: inability to purposefully move within physical environment (including bed mobility; transfer and ambulation); requires assistance; reluctance to attempt to move; limited range of motion; decreased muscle strength; decreased muscle control; imposed restrictions of movement (mechanical or medical protocol); impaired coordination; falling or stumbling; inflammation at site (redness, edema, tenderness); carries injured part protectively; muscle wasting

Pain

Definition: the state in which an individual experiences and reports the presence of severe discomfort or an uncomfortable sensation.

Related Factors
- Inflammatory process
- Muscle spasm
- Effects of trauma/surgery
- Immobility
- Pressure
- Infectious process
- Overactivity
- Ischemia
- Injuring agents (biologic, chemical, physical, psychologic)

Defining Characteristics
Subjective: verbal reports of pain, discomfort, anxiety, uncomfortable sensation.
Objective: guarding, limping, facial mask or grimace, increased respirations, increased heart rate, increased blood pressure, anxious, restlessness, nausea, vomiting, diaphoresis, moaning, crying, pacing, self focusing.

Self-care deficit (bathing, hygiene, dressing, grooming, feeding, toileting)

Definition: the state in which an individual experiences impaired ability independently to perform self-care activities

Related Factors
- Neuromuscular impairment
- Musculoskeletal impairment
- Cognitive impairment
- Sensory impairment
- Trauma
- Surgical procedures
- Restrictive devices
- Imposed restrictions
- Activity intolerance
- Pain/discomfort
- Ineffective coping with body change
- Depression
- Severe anxiety

Defining Characteristics
Subjective: verbal resports of difficulty performing daily activities.
Objective: partial or complete inability in performing desired activities.

Related Nursing Diagnoses
Activity intolerance
Body image disturbance
Chronic pain
Diversional activity deficit
Impaired home maintenance management
Impaired skin integrity
Sleep pattern disturbance
Fatigue
Altered role performance
Anxiety
High risk for disuse syndrome
High risk for trauma / injury
High risk for altered peripheral tissue perfusion
Knowledge deficit

CASE STUDY

Miss M. is a 72-year-old female who was brought to the emergency room with complaints of pain in the left hip and an inability to bear weight on the left leg.

Health History

Chielf complaint: inability to bear weight on the left leg and pain in the left hip area.

Present problem: the day of admission she slipped in the bath tub, fell on her left side and was unable to get up; complained of intense pain (10, on a scale of 1-10); ambulance was called by the neighbor, and patient was brought to the hospital.

Past medical history: diagnosed with arthritis in hands and wrists approximately 20 years ago; complains of stiffness and weakness in both hands with limited use; pneumonia 6 years ago; medications: aspirin 1/day; Motrin 400 mg tid (for pain in her hands).

Family history: both parents suffered from arthritis; parents died at an early age, reason unknown; no siblings.

Social history: walks 2 miles/day; able to perform all activities of daily living; tries to maintain a well-balanced diet.

Physical Examination

General: 72-year-old obese female: ht 5'6", wt 210 lb, BP 152/70, pulse 104, resp 28, temp 98.2° F.

Inspection: supine position with head of bed elevated 45 degrees; unable to stand or bear weight on left leg; left hip is swollen with areas of ecchymosis and bruising: no open areas noted; able to move left leg slightly with intense pain; generalized skin color pale, grimacing on face with frequent episodes of crying; left hip deformed and distal left leg externally rotated; restless and anxious; metacarpophalangeal and proximal interphalangeal joints englarged, both hands have no redness or angled deformities.

Palpation: left hip warm and tender to touch; bilateral pedal and popliteal pulses 1+; complains of slight tenderness during palpation of bilateral phalanges and wrist.

Muscle strength and range of motion (ROM): unable to assess full extent of ROM and muscle strength of left leg and hip due to intense pain with any movement; flexion and extension of bilateral phalanges slightly decreased; complains of stiffness and tenderness with movement; decreased strength in both hands (muscle strength = 3, symmetrically).

Diagnostic Tests

Left hip x-ray: oblique, displaced fracture of head of femur.

Problems identified for Miss M.

Pain (acute) related to soft tissue trauma and fracture
Defining Characteristics

Subjective: complains of pain in left hip with and without movement (10, scale 1-10).

Objective: left hip swollen; reluctance to move left leg; grimacing on face; episodes of crying; left hip deformed; left leg externally rotated; restless and anxious; increased heart rate; increased respirations; increased blood pressure.

Impaired physical mobility related to bone fracture and soft tissue trauma.
Defining Characteristics

Subjective: complains of intense pain with movement of left leg and hip; states unable to bear weight on left leg.

Objective: left hip area swollen with areas of ecchymosis and bruising; reluctance to move extremity; left hip deformed; left hip externally rotated.

Other problems to consider:

Self care deficit (bathing, hygiene, dressing, grooming, feeding, toileting related to hip fracture and pain)

Activity intolerance related to left hip fracture and pain.

Anxiety related to sudden, unexpected injury and loss of mobility.

Chronic pain related to joint stiffness and tenderness (bilaterial phalanges)

Knowledge deficit related to injury, trauma, and new equipment.

HEALTH PROMOTION

Risk factors associated with osteoporosis

- Race: white
- Blond or red hair, freckles
- Slight build, low weight
- Northwestern European descent
- Family history of osteoporosis
- Menopause before age 45
- Postmenopause
- Cigarette, heavy alcohol and caffeine use
- Sedentary life-style
- Scoliosis
- Hypermobility of joints
- Easy bruisability
- Poor dietary intake of calcium, vitamin D and protein
- Poor teeth
- Prolonged use of steroids, magnesium-based antacids and heparin

Ways to combat osteoporosis

- Consult your physician about estrogen replacement postmenopause
- Avoid cigarette smoking
- Avoid heavy use of alcohol and caffeine
- Include daily periods of exercise
- Increase dietary intake of calcium andvitamin D,
- Consult your physician about calcium and vitamin D supplements

Neurologic System and Mental Status

NURSING CONSIDERATIONS

Health History

While obtaining information for the health history, the nurse can be assessing the mental status of the patient. Areas include appearance, emotional stability, cognitive abilities, speech, and language. Use a systematic approach, progressing from general to specific questions, from nonthreatening to more threatening ones. Even though this health history focuses on the nervous system, use a holistic approach and inquire about the patient's general well-being and overall body function, including activities of daily living. Many nervous system disorders can cause or result from problems in other body systems. For example, a patient with a respiratory disorder that causes an impaired gas exchange can have affected cerebral function and neurologic symptoms. Serial evaluations of cognitive functions, especially level of consciousness, are recommended in patients with actual or potential alterations of cerebral structures and functions. This guards against relying on one assessment that may be made during the improvement or deterioration of a person's condition. Also, use good judgment when interpreting a person's statements about person, place, and time. Your patient may respond in a manner you deem inappropriate, when in fact, for them it is appropriate. For example, a patient who has been hospitalized for a lengthy time may become confused as to the day of the week, just as we often forget the date when writing a check. When evaluating mental status, it is important to consider the patient's culture, beliefs, fears regarding illness, family responsibilities, attitudes of others, financial worries, age, and intellectual status. For example, some proverbs may be culturally bound or more familiar to patients of a certain age group. Another example would be that in some Southeast Asian cultures, direct eye contact is avoided, especially by women, since the examiner is considered to hold a position of respect.

A patient's ability to detect environmental stimuli accurately directly influences orientation. Elderly patients often experience a decrease in visual and auditory acuity ,which may prevent them from properly recognizing or interpreting stimuli in the hospital environment. Also, the elderly patient may process information more slowly. Because of this, it may be necessary to repeat the question and allow adequate response time.

For a non-English speaking patient, a language barrier can cause an inaccurate assessment of the patient's orientation. Consult an interpreter and/or family and friends during your assessment. An aphasic patient may also seem disoriented, when in fact, the patient may not understand your questions. Remember that orientation actually reflects the patient's ability to correctly interpret and respond to his or her surroundings.

It is important to verify any critical or questionable information with another source, since a patient with a brain injury or disorder may have difficulty processing or recalling information. Other sources of information include family members, friends, and previous records. Because such a patient may tire easily, consider dividing the interview into several short sessions.

Physical Examination
Before beginning the physical examination, be mindful that some maneuvers may be difficult for your patient to perform, especially an elderly patient or one with a neurologic disorder affecting balance coordination. Be sensitive to your patient's condition and assess their ability to perform the maneuvers. When a patient does not do something you have instructed, you need to consider whether he understood the directions before determining he has a neurologic defect.

DIAGNOSTIC TESTS

X-ray (spinal): allows the visualization of the cervical, thoracic, lumbar and sacral regions of the spine; provides data primarily concerning injuries, fractures, dislocations, and other bony abnormalities.

X-ray (skull): allow for the visualization of the bones and nasal sinuses to identify fractures, tumors, vascular abnormalities, and cranial anomalies.

Computed tomography (CT): through the use of radiologic imaging and computer analysis, this test provides a three-dimensional view of the brain and spinal cord; these pictures aid in the detection and evaluation of tumors, trauma, abscesses, hemorrhages, and abnormal brain development.

Magnetic Resonance Imaging (MRI): provides images of body tissues that are used in the evaluation of cerebral infarctions, tumors, central nervous system (CNS) disorders such as congenital anomalies, and the condition of blood vessels and determining blood flow.

Lumbar puncture: done for several reasons: (1) to obtain and examine cerebrospinal fluid (CSF), (2) to determine the level of CSF pressure which aids in assessing CSF flow, and (3) to introduce anesthetics, drugs, and radiographic contrast media. This examination assists in the diagnosis of cerebral infections, hemorrhages, and metastatic changes.

Electromyography (EMG): measures nerve conduction and electrical properties of skeletal muscles; it is done to detect neuromuscular abnormalities.

Electroencephalography (EEG): measures and records electrical impulses from the cortex of the brain; it provides diagnostic data about abnormal electrical activity in the brain and aids in the diagnosis of such disorders as epilepsy, brain tumors, hematomas, drug intoxication, cerebral blood flow disorder, and cerebrovascular diseases.

Cerebral angiography: an injection of radiopague dye, this test allows for radiographic visualization of the cerebral vascular system; provides information about the patency, size, irregularities, or occlusion of the cerebral vessels.

Myelography (myelogram): uses a radiopaque solution, injected into the spinal canal which allows visualization of the contents of the spinal canal; used to evaluate intervertebral disk integrity or herniation, the presence of tumors, spinal obstruction, or the existence of developmental or degenerative spinal conditions.

NURSING DIAGNOSES

Altered thought processes
Definition: the state in which an individual experiences a disruption in cognitive operations and activities.

Related Factors

- Side effects of sedatives, narcotics, or anesthetics
- Altered biochemistry
- Cerebral hypoxia
- Fever or hypothermia
- Effects of aging
- Physiologic changes
- Psychologic conflicts
- Loss of memory
- Impaired judgment
- Altered sensory input (overload/deprivation)
- Immobility
- Sleep deprivation
- Caloric deprivation
- Depression
- Pain
- Anxiety/stress
- Fear of the unknown
- Actual loss of: control/familiar objects/routine surroundings/income/significant other
- Social isolation

Defining Characteristics

Subjective: verbal reports of difficulties thinking and focusing; complains of being distracted; verbalizes periodic loss of memory; forgetting things; difficulty with ideas of reference; verbalizes hallucinations and delusions.

Objective: impaired ability to abstract or conceptualize; impaired ability to calculate; altered attention span; obsessions; inability to follow commands; disorientation to time/place/person/circumstances/events; changes in remote, recent and/or immediate memory; delusions; hallucinations; inappropriate social behavior; inappropriate affect; combative/agitated behavior; inability to solve problems; sundowning(onset of confusion at end of day); frightened/unsafe behavior (climbing out of bed, removing tubes); decreased ability to grasp ideas; nonsensical speech; egocentricity.

Altered tissue perfusion (cerebral)

Definition: the state in which an individual experiences a decrease in nutrition or oxygenation at the cellular level due to a deficit in capillary blood supply.

Related Factors

- Interruption of arterial flow
- Interruption of venous flow
- Hypervolemia
- Hypovolemia
- Trauma
- Prolonged sitting/standing
- Immobilization
- Oxygen/carbon dioxide exchange problems
- Decreased cardiac output
- Increased peripheral vascular resistance

Defining Characteristics

Subjective: verbal reports of difficulties with memory.

Objective: alteration in thought processes, restlessness, altered consciousness, memory loss, confusion, blurred vision, syncope/vertigo, unequal or dilated pupils.

Impaired communication (verbal and/or nonverbal)

Definition: the state in which an individual experiences a decreased or absent ability to use or understand language in human interaction.

Related Factors

- Decrease in circulation to brain
- Effects of surgery/trauma
- Compromised respiratory efforts
- Ineffective listening skills
- Physical barriers (brain tumor, tracheostomy, intubation)
- Anatomic deficit
- Psychological barriers
- Cultural differences
- Developmental or age related
- Administration of central nervous system depressants
- Disorientation
- Dysarthria
- Aphasia
- Fatigue
- Hearing impairment
- Language barriers

Defining Characteristics

Subjective: verbal reports of difficulty in expressing thoughts; indicates a weak or absent voice; reports difficulty in expressing self; indicates lack of comprehension of understanding of spoken words.

Objective: inability to speak dominant language; refusal or inability to speak; stuttering; slurring; impaired articulation; disorientation; inability to modulate speech; flight of ideas; incessant verbalization; difficulty with phonation; inability to speak in sentences; inappropriate speech; exhibiting frustration/anger while trying to express self or understand someone else; presence of barrier preventing communication (tracheostomy, endotracheal tube).

Sensory-perceptual alterations (kinesthetic, tactile)

Definition: a state in which an individual experiences interruption or change in reception and/or interpretation of stimuli by receptors for body position or touch.

Related Factors

- Kinesthetic

  Effects of inner ear inflammation

  Neurological impairment (disease, trauma, deficit)

  Side effects of tranquilizers, sedatives, muscle relaxants, or antihistamines

  Sleep deprivation

  Pain (phantom limb)

- Tactile

  Circulatory impairment (disease, trauma, deficit)

  Inflammation

  Effects of anesthesia

  Nutritional deficiencies

  Effects of aging

  Effects of burns

  Neurological impairment

  Pain

  Persistent tactile stimulation

Defining Characteristics

Kinesthetic

Subjective: verbal reports of nausea; inability to tell position of body parts (proprioception); vertigo.
Objective: falling; stumbling; alteration in posture; inability to sit or stand.

Tactile

Subjective: verbal reports of change in sensory status: hypo/hyper peresthesias
Objective: measured changes in sensory status: paresthesias, hyperesthesias, anesthesias

High risk for injury

Definition: the state in which an individual is at risk of injury as a result of environmental conditions interacting with the individual's adaptive and defensive resources.

Risk Factors
Internal
Biochemical
Regulatory function: sensory, integrative, effector dysfunction
Tissue hypoxia
Malnutrition
Abnormal blood profile: leukocytosis or leukopenia, altered clotting factors, thrombocytopenia, sickle cell, decreased hemoglobin level
Physical
Broken skin
Altered mobility
Developmental
Age (physiologic, psychosocial)
Psychologic
Affective
Orientation

Biologic
Immunization level of community
Microorganism
Chemical
Poisons
Drugs: pharmaceutical agents, alcohol, caffeine, nicotine
Preservatives
Physical
Design, structure, and arrangement of community, building, and/or equipment
Mode of transport/transportation
Nosocomial agents
People-provider
Nosocomial agents
Staffing patterns
Cognitive, affective, and psychomotor factors

External

Defining Characteristics
Subjective: may report loss of memory; lack of concentration; confusion, disorientation, decreased problem-solving ability, difficulty with balance, problems moving arms or walking; problems with speech; having a seizure, or getting lost.
Objective: impaired memory; short attention span; distractibility; impaired judgment; agitation; hostile or combative behavior; impaired problem solving; unsteady gait; paralysis or paresis; sensory impairments; impaired speech; seizures; wandering and/or falling.

Related Nursing Diagnoses
Ineffective breathing pattern
Impaired physical mobility
Altered urinary elimination
Altered bowel elimination
Altered nutrition: less than body requirements
Total/partial self-care deficit
Altered sexuality patterns
Social isolation
Altered family processes
Body image disturbance
Anticipatory grieving
Anxiety
High risk for impaired adjustment
Self-esteem disturbance
Powerlessness
Ineffective individual/family coping
Hopelessness
Altered health maintenance
Knowledge deficit

CASE STUDY

Mr. K. is a 62-year-old white male office manager, admitted to the hospital complaining of a severe headache and not being able to move his left side (arm and leg).

Health History

Chief complaint: complains of a severe headache and not being able to move his left side.

Present problem: was grocery shopping when he suddenly passed out; he awoke approximately 5 minutes later complaining of a severe headache and not being able to move his left arm and leg; an ambulance then brought him to the hospital; slight facial droop noted left side of face with some slurring of speech.

Past medical history: diagnosed with hypertension approximately 7 years ago (partially controlled with medication); myocardial infarction 3 years ago.

Family history: father died of heart disease at age 52; mother living and well; brother diagnosed with hypertension at age 42.

Social history: smokes cigarettes 1 pack/day x 15 years; has sedentary lifestyle; eats a regular diet.

Physical Examination

General: 62-year-old male: ht 5'11", wt 228 lbs, BP 162/90, pulse 92, resp 22, temp 98.4 F.

Cerebral status **(mental status):** appearance, behavior, and speech appropriate; alert and oriented x3; slightly anxious concerning present condition; body language and facial expression appropriate; recent and remote memory intact.

Cranial Nerves:

  I Identifies coffee and alcohol appropriately

  II Vision 20/20; peripheral fields intact by confrontation; fundi within normal limits

  III 6 cardinal fields of gaze intact; PERRLA bilateral

  IV See III

  V Decreased sharp and dull sensations noted on left side of face; jaw strength decreased, left side of face; inability to chew on left side.

  VI See II

  VII Motor weakness noted left side of face, unable to smile on left side.

  VIII Hearing intact bilaterally

  IX Swallowing intact; gag reflex present; uvular rises midline on phonation

  X See IX

  XII Tongue protrudes midline; no tremors

Cerebellar status **(motor status):** left hand grasp weak; unable to perform purposeful movement of left arm; left leg weak; unable to support weight; has full range-of-motion (passive on left side only); finger to nose smoothly intact right side only.

Sensory status: superficial pain and light touch sensation not detected on left side; vibration intact bilateral; position sense intact on right side but impaired on left side; stereognosis intact bilateral.

Reflexes: all deep tendon reflexes intact bilaterally; plantar reflex negative.

Diagnostic Tests

Skull x-ray: intracranial calcifications, hemorrhage

Computed tomography: intracerebral hemorrhage

Cerebral angiography: shows narrowing of large vessels

Magnetic resonance imaging: intracerebral hemorrhage

Electroencephalography: shows focal slowing around area of lesion

Problems identified for Mr. K.

Impaired physical mobility related to neurovascular impairment

Defining Characteristics

Subjective: complains of not being able to move left arm and leg; verbalizes not being able to chew on the left side.

Objective: unable to perform purposeful movement of left arm and leg; left hand grasp weak; left leg weak; unable to support weight; jaw strength decreased left side of face; skull x-ray, computed tomography, magnetic resonance imaging show intracerebral hemorrhage; absence of smile on left side; ptosis and flat nasolabial folds on left side of face.

Sensory/perceptual alteration related to neurovascular impairment.

Defining Characteristics

Subjective: states he is unable to feel pin prick or light touch on left side of face, left arm and left leg.

Objective: superficial pain and light touch sensation not detected on left side; position sense impaired on left side.

Self-care deficit related to sensory and motor deficit

Defining Characteristics

Subjective: verbalizes inability to move left arm and leg.

Objective: impaired ability to bathe, dress, groom, feed, and toilet self; unable to perform purposeful movements with left arm; unable to support weight; inability to perform active range-of-motion on left side; impaired position sense left side; superficial pain and light touch sensation not detect on left side.

High risk for injury related to impaired sensory and motor function

Defining Characteristics

Subjective: complains of not being able to move left arm and leg; verbalizes a lack of feeling in left arm and leg.

Objective: decreased motor function in left arm and leg; decreased sensory status in left arm and leg; unable to perform purposeful movement with left arm; unable to support weight; position sense impaired on left side.

Other problems to consider

Body image disturbance related to loss of body function and inability to perform self-care

Anxiety related to present condition and new surroundings

High risk for impaired skin integrity

High risk for anticipatory grieving

High risk for self-esteem disturbance

High risk for altered sexuality patterns or sexual dysfunction

HEALTH PROMOTION

Risk factors associated with cerebrovascular accidents

- Hypertension
- Obesity
- Sedentary life-style
- Smoking tobacco products
- Stress Increased level of serum cholesterol, lipoproteins, and triglycerides
- Use of oral contraceptives in high-risk women
- Family history of diabetes mellitus, cardiovascular disease, hypertension, and increased serum cholesterol levels
- Congenital cerebrovascular anomalies (taken directly from textbook)

Precautions for persons with confusion or impaired judgment
- Keep living area clutter free
- Avoid frequent rearranging of surroundings
- Remove throw rugs to avoid slipping
- Remove breakables and dangerous items (matches, knives, guns, poisons)
- Keep medications in locked cabinet or drawer
- Keep doors locked to potentially dangerous areas (basements)
- Keep exit doors locked and install door alarms, if person has a tendency to wander
- Have the person wear or carry some sort of identification
- Make sure clothing fits properly and shoes have nonskid soles
- Utilize night-lights to help prevent falls
- Have the person attended in seems confused or agitated
- Encourage frequent rest periods throughout the day to avoid being overtired
- Provide clothing appropriate for the season
- Keep person's bed in low position
- Install side rails to bed if person is at risk for falling

Things to avoid for a confused person
- Alcohol
- Contact sports
- Swimming without supervision
- Hunting
- Power tools or sharp implements
- Driving
- Cooking without supervision

References

Canobbio M: *Cardiovascular disorders*, St Louis, 1990, Mosby.

Mourad L: *Orthopedic disorders*, St Louis, 1991, Mosby.

Brundage D: *Renal disorders*, St Louis, 1992, Mosby.

Chips E, Clanin N, Campbell V: *Neurologic disorders*, St Louis, 1990, Mosby.

Wilson S, Thompson J: *Respiratory disorders*, St Louis, 1990, Mosby.

Morton P: *Health assessment in nursing*, ed 2, Philadelphia, 1993, Springhouse Corporation.

Seidel H, Ball J, Dains J, Benedict G: *Mosby's guide to physical examination*, ed 2, St Louis, 1991, Mosby.

Fuller J, Schaller-Ayers J: *Health assessment - a nursing approach*, ed 2, Philadelphia, 1994, Lippincott.

Jarvis C: *Physical examination and health assessment*, Philadelphia, 1992, Saunders.

Barkauskas V, Stoltenberg-Allen K, Baumann L, Darling-Fisher C: *Health and physical assessment*, St Louis, 1994, Mosby.

Fischbach F: *A manual of laboratory and diagnostic tests*, ed 4, Philadelphia, 1992, Lippincott.

Pagana K, Pagana T: Mosby's diagnostic and laboratory test reference, St Louis, 1992, Mosby.

Kim M, McFarland G, McLane A: Pocket guide to nursing diagnosis, ed 5, St Louis, 1993, Mosby.

Taptich B, Iyer P, Bernocchi-Losey D: *Nursing diagnosis and care planning*, Philadelphia, 1989, Saunders.

Doenges M, Moorhouse M: *Application of nursing process and nursing diagnosis: an interactive text*, Philadelphia, 1992, FA Davis.

Lueckenotte A: *Pocket guide to gerontologic assessment*, ed 2, St Louis, 1994, Mosby.

Lewis S, Collier I: *Medical-surgical nursing - assessment and management of clinical problems*, ed 3, St Louis, 1992, Mosby.

Phipps W, Long B, Woods N, Cassmeyer V: *Medical-surgical nursing - concepts and clinical practice*, ed 4, St Louis, 1991, Mosby.

Seidel Textbook Page Numbers

Corresponding to Learning Activities Questions

Chapter 1

1-4	p. 2
5-6	pp. 3-7
7-11	pp. 8-10
12-14	pp. 11-13
15	p. 15
16	p. 4
17	p. 11
18	pp. 3-4
19	p. 5
20-21	p. 8
22	p. 5
23-27	pp. 14-15
28	p. 16
29	p. 27
30	p. 12
31	p. 15
32	p. 16
33	pp. 17-18
34	p. 18
35	p. 21
36	pp. 22-23
37	pp. 24-25
38	p. 29
39	p. 31
40	p. 32
41-60	(See Part II)*

Chapter 2

1-5	pp. 34-36
6-18	p. 36
19-21	pp. 37-38
22-33	p. 39
34-40	pp. 40-44
41-46	pp. 46-51
47	pp. 52-53
48	p. 53
49-58	pp. 54-56
59-60	p. 56

Chapter 3

1-10	pp. 57-61
11-23	p. 61
24-25	pp. 57-58, 62
26	p. 57
27	pp. 58-59
28	p. 60
29	pp. 61-62
30	pp. 57-60
31	p. 64

32	p. 65
33	p. 68
34	p. 64
35	p. 65
36	pp. 70-71
37	p. 71
38	p. 72
39	p. 75
40	p. 76
41	p. 77
42	p. 78
43	p. 80
44	p. 82
45-48	p. 71
49-52	p. 77
53-56	pp. 76, 79, 81-82
57-60	pp. 74-75, 79-80

Chapter 4

1	p. 84
2	pp. 84-85
3	pp. 86-87
4-5	p. 87
6	p. 88
7-10	p. 89
11-21	pp. 90-91
22	pp. 95-96
23	pp. 92, 94
24	pp. 108-109
25-28	pp. 104-107
29	p. 90
30-31	p. 92
32	p. 95
33	p. 96
34	p. 98
35	p. 107
36	pp. 109, 117
37	p. 117
38	p. 118
39	pp. 118-121
40	p. 126
41-47	pp. 125-129
48-50	p. 92 (See Part II)*

*Nursing Considerations content in Part II of this workbook.

Chapter 5

Chapter 6

Chapter 7

Chapter 20

1-3	pp. 807, 811, 814-815
4-7	pp. 811-815
8	p. 807
9	pp. 811-812
10-11	p. 812
12	p. 815
13-17	pp. 808-810
18	p. 813
19	pp. 814-815
20-21	p. 815
22	p. 816
23	p. 808
24	p. 809
25	p. 816
26	p. 817
27	pp. 818-819
28	p. 819
29	p. 824
30	p. 825
31	p. 826
32	p. 827
33-40	p. 823

Chapter 21

1	p. 828
2-7	pp. 828-831
8	p. 832
9	p. 833
10	p. 832
11	p. 833
12	p. 834
13	pp. 839-840
14	p. 840
15-34	pp. 832-837
35-51	pp. 837-839
52	pp. 841-842
53-54	pp. 842-843
55	p. 844
56	p. 845
57	p. 847
58	p. 848
59	p. 850
60	p. 851

STUDENT WORKBOOK
to accompany

Mosby's Guide to

PHYSICAL
EXAMINATION